Reiki for Dogs

Reiki for Dogs

Using Spiritual Energy to Heal and Vitalize
Man's Best Friend

Kathleen Prasad

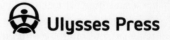 Ulysses Press

Published in the United States by
Ulysses Press
P.O. Box 3440
Berkeley, CA 94703
www.ulyssespress.com

ISBN13: 978-1-61243-048-5
Library of Congress Control Number 2012931430

Printed in Canada by Webcom

10 9 8 7 6 5 4 3 2 1

Acquisitions Editor: Keith Riegert
Managing Editor: Claire Chun
Editor: Nicky Leach
Proofreader: Lauren Harrison
Production: Abby Reser, Judith Metzener
Index: Sayre Van Young
Cover design: what!design @ whatweb.com
Interior and back cover photographs: © Lexie Cataldo
    (www.injoyphotography.com)
Front cover photographs: top © Kendra Luck (www.dogumentarian.com);
    bottom © Raywoo/shutterstock.com

Distributed by Publishers Group West

DISCLAIMER: The suggestions in this book are not intended as a substitute for professional veterinary care. Reiki sessions are given for the purpose of stress reduction and relaxation to promote healing. Reiki is not a substitute for medical diagnosis and treatment. Reiki practitioners do not diagnose conditions nor do they prescribe, perform medical treatment, nor interfere with the treatment of a licensed medical professional. It is recommended that animals be taken to a licensed veterinarian or licensed health care professional for any ailment they have.

For my little rainbow fairy, Indigo.

Table of Contents

Muffet, Dakota, and Mystic—The Forever Dogs of My Heart

When I was little, I was tremendously shy. I spent lots of time alone. Even from an early age, animals appealed to me more than people. I just understood them better, trusted them more.

My best friend growing up was a sheltie/collie mix named Muffet. Most of my childhood memories involve her. She's in my lap in many of the photos of my early years. I remember her comforting presence during both good and bad times as I grew. She was incredibly sensitive and gentle, and being a herding breed, she was always at my side. It's because of her that I came to love dogs so much, and rely upon their constant presence. She passed away the year I went away to college, but she will always be a part of who I am.

My Shadow

Dakota came into my life after college when I was a single young adult. I adopted him from county animal control when he was just a three-month-old puppy. He followed me through many life changes, including various moves, starting my teaching career, getting married, and eventually adding our daughter to the family. He was the first animal I ever tried to offer Reiki to, thus I consider him my first animal Reiki teacher. He showed me so much about what energetic connections between dogs and people could be, what communication between species could look like. He was with me on this earth, at my side, for 16 years, and our spirits will always be connected. Dakota was a dog with a heart of gold, a wisdom beyond his years, and a soul that touched everyone who met him.

Now as I walk through my adult life, day in and day out, my shadow is never alone. At my left side there is another shadow attached to my own form. You won't see this if you look with your eyes, but look deeper with your heart and I think you will. There he is, my Aussie mix, his fuzzy, lithe body prancing every step, the end of his tail turned up just a little bit. Dakota's spirit always follows me, right at my ankle. He may physically be gone from this planet, but still his energy remains with me.

Surviving

After Dakota passed, my world went dark for a long time. I shed more tears than I can count. Even with all the Reiki in the world, a grief passed through my heart so deeply that it has forever changed me. I used to wonder, could I ever love another dog after Dakota? Honestly, I thought, maybe my heart was just too broken.

After about three years, I just couldn't stand being without a dog in the house anymore so, with my husband's blessing, I started to look for our new family member. My husband left it up to me. "Let Reiki help you find our new dog," he said. In my heart, I also asked Dakota to help me find the right dog. Each time I would go see a potential dog to adopt, I would meditate and open my heart. "Show me a sign." I knew my heart would know when I saw the right one.

Finding the One to Rescue

Many rescued puppies and dogs passed my way. One was even named Dakota and had blue eyes just like our dearest departed. But none could move me. My heart was completely still, no matter how cute, how lovable the puppy was.

Then one day, my sister found a tiny six-week-old border collie/Catahoula mix on petfinder.com. The pregnant mother of this puppy was rescued at the last minute from the euthanasia list at a Utah shelter, and somehow she ended up at a nearby California rescue group with her nine puppies. Something about the photo of one little puppy's face in particular made me go for a visit.

As I held her little four-pound body in my arms, she leaned into my chest, her tail wagging furiously. And all at once, my heart that had been silent as a stone for so long suddenly expanded out of my chest. It was as if my heart came back to life—as if I already loved her, somehow, even though I had never met her before. I was overwhelmed. Her tail continued to wag and wag, moving faster each time I spoke to her. She snuggled into my neck and whined ever so slightly. That was it, I knew without a doubt, she was the one!

Sure enough, she won over my four-year-old daughter and my husband immediately. She seemed the perfect fit for our family: loving, gentle, silly, and she even had gray fur and blue eyes (as if in tribute to our dear Dakota). On our first vet's appointment, we discovered that she is blind in one eye—most likely a congenital defect. No worries, she is still perfect to us. After all, sometimes we can see more clearly with our hearts than our eyes anyway. In honor of her spirit, we dubbed her Mystic. What a beautiful light she brings to our home!

Saving Me

Less than two months later, when Mystic was a mere three months old, I was holding her to my chest, and she began scratching me. I put her down and reached up ("Ouch!") to feel my chest. It was then that I unexpectedly felt a lump in my left breast. Several scans and a biopsy revealed that it was, indeed, breast cancer. Aged just 41, I couldn't believe it. This was truly a shock to me.

As I write these words, I am only a month out of surgery, recovering and getting stronger every day. Thank goodness it was detected early and has not spread, so I am expected to recover fully without any further treatment. I feel so blessed to live each day with my family, friends, and animals. Life has never tasted sweeter, truly. And little did I know when I picked up that tiny little puppy that needed rescuing that she actually might be the one who would save my life. Life is funny sometimes, isn't it?

And through it all, Muffet and Dakota are still with me—yes, I feel their presence. Our dogs touch our lives so deeply; they are always with us, not only when they are in their bodies running by our sides but also when they move into spirit and wrap themselves around our hearts for eternity. I dedicate this book to the forever dogs of my heart: Muffet, Dakota, and Mystic.

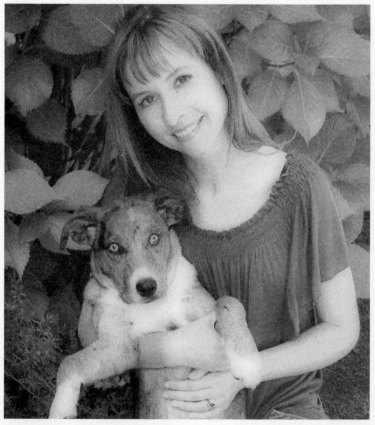

Author Kathleen Prasad with Mystic.

May reading this book bring to mind a lifetime of memories of your own forever dogs of the heart. May your spirit be light with the memories of golden moments together. And may reading this book help support you in finding a deeper spiritual bond with the dog you share your life with now, and with those dogs yet to find you.

PART I
The Foundation

I come to realize that mind is no other than mountains and rivers and the great wide earth, the sun, and the moon and stars.

—Dogen

CHAPTER 1

Reiki to the Rescue!

The quieter you become, the more you can hear.
—Baba Ram Dass

We've all been there at one time or another. Unexpectedly, our beloved dog is injured, and we wish we could help. A stray dog wanders by our property, limping, and we think if only we could do something. The neighbor's dog is diagnosed with cancer, and we feel bad for them but helpless. Our dog is sick, and on the way to the vet we lament that there is nothing we can do in the meantime. We can't even visit our local animal shelter because we can't take them *all* home. And, most painfully, we hold our beloved canine companion in our arms as they die and wish with all our hearts that we could somehow ease the transition.

But what if you *could* do something? What if you could safely and effectively help in all these situations? What if there were something you could do that would be helpful and healing for all dogs, all the time?

I am here to tell you, with certainty, that you *can* do something! With just a little practice, you can do it easily and always for the highest good of the dog and the situation. You can do it without fear of doing harm. You can do it simply, with your dedicated focus and intention. It isn't something magical or only for the gifted and talented few. It's your birth-right, your inner power and truth, your very essence. It's Reiki. Reiki to the rescue!

Opening the Door of Healing Possibility

I believe we are stewards of the animals on this planet. Because they cannot tell us in words what is wrong, why something hurts, or why they are anxious, we must learn to listen to their nonverbal cues in order to understand them. Anyone who has ever had a beloved companion animal knows what I'm talking about—that certain look your bird gives you, the nudge from your dog, the special meow from your cat, the snort from your horse. When you know an animal well, you begin to be able to read their subtle physical cues to determine what is going on with them. On a deeper level, you can often sense what is going on with them emotionally or when something is "off."

With Reiki, you make profound and deep connections with your animal that allow you to sometimes understand more completely what he or she is going through. In this book, we will explore, in particular, the profound and deep connec-tions we can make with our dogs through energy work.

I remember a particular dog that I worked with at the animal shelter. He was extremely timid and fearful of humans, shunning all contact with them, especially when they came into his kennel. As I offered Reiki, I had a sudden vision of a human kicking this little dog over and over. In the space of energetic Reiki connection, the little doggie had shared this memory with me. As I continued to offer Reiki, the little dog slowly came over to me, crawled into my lap, and fell into a peaceful sleep. I realized that Reiki was not only helping the dog to release his painful past, but also that in my very action of offering this healing to him he now had a positive human experience upon which to build a future of trust.

Your trusted vet may be able to diagnose what is physically wrong with your dog. And you may have a sense of what is emotionally wrong, based upon the dog's past—perhaps, for example, you have adopted a dog that you know was formerly

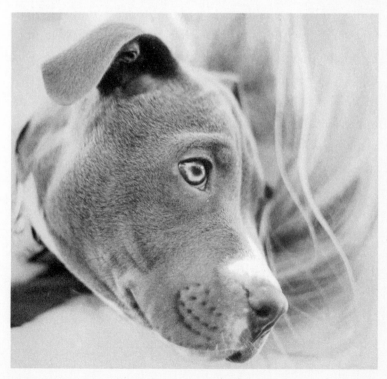

beaten, abused, or abandoned by her previous humans. But even when you have an idea of what the problem is, you may often feel helpless about how to address these issues, which originate in the past.

Sometimes you don't know anything about the background of the dog you have adopted, and you can only guess at possibilities based upon the dog's behaviors. Or you may have raised your dog since the day he or she was born, and it may just be that they have a highly stressed personality type or a particular genetic physical problem.

The wonderful thing about Reiki is that you can offer healing to your dog without having to know what is wrong. Although it is valuable and important to have your veterinarian working with you to help your dog, you don't have to sit by, unable to assist. Whatever the issues your dogs face, with Reiki, you never have to feel powerless again. Reiki is a way to support balance, healing, peace, and harmony for all situations—physical, mental, emotional, and spiritual. Even more amazing, sometimes your dogs might even tell you exactly where they hurt!

It's good to remember, too, that your dogs are part of your family, and when one member of the family is sick, injured, or stressed, everyone in the family is affected. When you are sick your dogs worry about you, sometimes even taking on your problems to help you. When your dogs are sick, you worry. And when one dog is sick, the other dogs in your family know and are concerned and affected. Reiki is a way to support the whole family in times of health challenges and/or crisis.

Perhaps your dogs have lived a beautiful life with you from babyhood to senior years, but they are in their end stage of life. Whether your dog is in good health and winding down gracefully or fighting chronic disease or cancer, you can see death approaching, and you feel powerless.

Over many years of working with the animals in hospice at BrightHaven, a holistic animal retreat that serves senior and special-needs animals in picturesque Sonoma County, California, I have been amazed to witness how Reiki brings peace and healing as the animals approach their transitions. The change is profound. The animals come forward and literally "ask" for Reiki, understanding that it can help them at the end of life.

The Key

Reiki is not a magic spell. It's not something you "give" to someone else. Reiki is about connection and balance on the most elemental levels of your spirit. Reiki is part of your essence—underneath it all, if you could see into your very soul, it *is* who you are. All you need to begin this journey are two things: your intention to offer this healing connection and your dog's acceptance of your offering. With those simple two ingredients, you can unlock the door of healing possibility in your life. What awaits you as you walk through that door is a universe of new depth and possibilities—a deeper awareness of the wisdom and beauty of dogs, which has always existed but remained unnoticed. Once you have connected with your dog in the beautiful, peaceful, healing space that is Reiki, your eyes will be forever opened to this new reality. Your life will be transformed—your bond with each other profoundly deepened.

CHAPTER 2

The Spiritual Wisdom of Dogs

Every animal knows more than you do.
—Native American proverb

To get the most out of our experiences with Reiki and dogs, it is helpful to consider the spiritual qualities of our dogs and what we can learn from them. When we share our lives with dogs, our spiritual paths intertwine. We are (consciously or unconsciously) changed for the better. Dogs are not only our closest companions and friends; they are also amazing spiritual teachers, simply because of the spiritual qualities they possess.

The most compassionate, forgiving, and loving beings I have known have been dogs. Dogs live selflessly and generously, with faithful, loyal, and trusting hearts. They bless us with their unconditional love and unending devotion. Dogs can be simultaneously gentle as lambs, yet fiercely protective of the ones they love. They know how to walk the line between martial courage and peaceful surrender. Dogs also sense and understand the subtlest of energetic vibrations.

Spending time with dogs can help us develop our own sensitivities. Dogs authentically embody so many spiritual qualities throughout their lives and even as they face death. Living with and loving dogs, we can be guided toward being better people and creating a healthier planet, one where people practice compassionate devotion and a life of joyful service to others.

Dogs as Mirrors

Think of the qualities of the dog or dogs in your life. Wise protector? Constant companion? Playful, silly puppy? The qualities your dog displays will point to areas where you need to develop your own inner qualities and heal yourself. Dogs can be mirrors of our inner selves, highlighting our strengths and challenges. If we can open up to this possibility we can see into our own hearts more easily and develop our highest and best qualities while healing our deepest issues. Dogs are truly our guides and teachers.

Dogs as Healers

Dogs have been associated with healing throughout history, and the psychological healing and support provided by service dogs of all kinds is today well-known. Take the example of Guide Dogs for the Blind. Not only is the guide dog the eyes for the blind person but he or she also serves as best friend, trusted guide, and loyal companion. Truly, all dogs—not just service dogs—provide healing. And in return for a lifetime of love, devotion, and service, what do our dogs require of us?

Really, nothing—although they do appreciate love and devotion, food, and a bit of play, silliness, and adventure. In so many ways and on so many levels, dogs bring so much to this world and to our lives. What better way to repay them for all they have given us than by offering Reiki back to them?

Animals as Reiki Teachers

When I began this journey with Reiki, I never imagined that I would find my focus with animals rather than people. But with each passing day, it seemed that more and more animals came my way in need of healing work.

In the early years, I kept a journal of the amazing experiences and lessons I learned through offering animals Reiki treatments. Many of these stories can be found in my first book, *Animal Reiki*. As time progressed, it was as if the animals that I worked with were asking me to be their voice—to

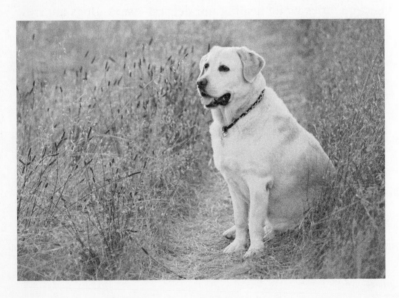

share what I had learned from them with other people, so that even more animals could be helped.

I found myself moving toward teaching Reiki for animals. At that time, this was something that really wasn't "done" in the Reiki community. Most practitioners specialized in working with people and just did Reiki treatments with animals here and there. So I asked the animals themselves for their help, advice, and wisdom—all the while continuing to practice, write about, and contemplate each experience I had doing Reiki with animals.

Over the years, the animals have shown me so much about the nature of energy and how we can more successfully commune with other species on the soul level. I feel so blessed to have had all these amazing animal teachers in my life. I hope some of the stories I share in this book inspire you to take a new and deeper look at the animals in your life!

CHAPTER 3

What Is Reiki?

And the end of all our exploring will be to arrive where
we started and know the place for the first time.
—T. S. Eliot

In classes, I often get asked what the word *Reiki* means. There are two ways to answer this question. First, let's look at the meaning of the word itself.

The word Reiki comes from two *kanji*, or Japanese characters used in writing: *Rei* ("spirit") and *Ki* ("energy"), so literally the Japanese word *Reiki* means "spiritual energy." This spiritual energy refers to the substance that forms all things—those little energetic particles that physicists have discovered make up solids, liquids, and air. When looking at the world through the energy lens, we see that all things are connected, all things are one, because all things are in essence part of the same substance: Reiki.

The defining quality of Reiki as an energetic pattern running through existence is balance through change. You can understand this essential truth best by watching the patterns of nature moving over time. This is Reiki in action. For instance, watching the waves crashing on the shore and the tide moving in and out is a powerful example of Reiki at work. So too are constantly shifting weather patterns, the cycle of the seasons, trees changing as they grow, flowers blooming and fading. The life cycles of all living beings, in fact, are physical, observable examples of Reiki, and Reiki is the language of nature.

The System of Reiki

The second use of the word Reiki is to describe a Japanese energy healing system that was originally used to assist spiritual development in Japan but today is most commonly used throughout the world for "hands-on" healing.

This system was developed by Mikao Usui, who lived in the late nineteenth and early twentieth centuries. Little is known about Mikao Usui's personal life. What we do know is this: He was born into a Hatamoto Samurai family (a high level of Samurai) and studied as a child in a Tendai Buddhist Monastery. He began studying martial arts at age 12 and gained the highest proficiency in weaponry and grappling.

After a varied career that took him to many countries, Usui eventually opened a Center of Usui Hands-On Healing, the aim of which was to achieve enlightenment. This was not a religion; there was no belief system attached. Usui used "attunements" (the ceremonial passing on of Reiki information from master to student) only to remind students of their spiritual connection. He also integrated mantras and meditations into his teachings. Hand positions and symbols were added to his system later to help students who had difficulty sensing the energy.

Over time, the practices and teachings of Reiki have evolved to reflect the people who teach Reiki. For example, my classes emphasize animal Reiki. Today, there are many lineages and branches of Reiki, each with its own teachings and emphasis. Keep in mind that Reiki is energetic in essence, and although these individual humanistic differences are interesting, they do not affect the inherent healing power that is Reiki. In other words, Reiki is beyond us and bigger than us; it is the very energetic essence of the universe, present in and all around us.

The Basics of the Reiki System

The system of Reiki has five elements, which, when used together, produce a powerful deepening of our connection to and awareness of the spiritual energy of the universe, or Reiki. Those of us who use the system of Reiki are called "practitioners," not "healers," since we do not manipulate the energy or healing of others. Through our compassionate intention, we simply open more deeply to the universal flow of energy, creating an "energetic space of healing," and in so doing, facilitate the healing process of others. Reiki can do no harm and is supportive of all other healing modalities and therapies, both allopathic and holistic.

As defined by world-renowned Reiki researchers and teachers Frans and Bronwen Stiene, founders of the International House of Reiki, the five elements of the system of Reiki are:

1. The Five Precepts, or Rules of Conduct
   For today only:
   - Do not anger
   - Do not worry
   - Be humble
   - Be honest in your work
   - Be compassionate to yourself and others
2. The Initiations (also called attunements, or *Reiju*)
3. Healing Practice
4. Symbols and Mantras
5. Traditional Techniques and Meditations

The system of Reiki is considered a practice. That means that your intention and commitment to the "doing" of Reiki is important to your own development, healing, and understanding of the healing process, as well as your ability to facilitate more energetic flow through your physical being. This practice never ends; it is a lifelong journey of self-discovery. The more you work with Reiki, the more you will open to this flow. For this reason, practicing Reiki can deepen your intuition and cause tremendous growth and change on all levels. Ideally, practitioners should be doing daily personal Reiki meditation and self-healing in addition to using Reiki with others.

The system of Reiki is holistic. It can be used for physical, mental, emotional, and spiritual healing. The nature of Reiki is harmony and balance, so it always finds the origin of health problems ("dis-ease," or imbalance) and works for the highest good (rebalancing and clearing the energy "flow"). Reiki cannot be forced upon another individual or animal; it will only flow according to the openness of the individual. In other words, each individual is responsible for his or her own healing process. What a practitioner does is simply, through practice, to learn how to create and hold a healing space to support another being.

To learn all of these elements is beyond the scope of this book: You would need to study with a Reiki teacher who can offer you energetic guidance and practice in each element. In searching for Reiki teachers to guide your own practice and healing journey, it is best to find teachers who resonate with your inner truth and support you with compassion and courage in following your unique soul's path. You may find that it's not only people but also dogs in your life who become your teachers in this journey.

This book will give you many exercises with which to begin your journey. Some of the Try This exercises in this book are traditional Reiki exercises and are labeled as such; other Try This exercises are meditative techniques I have created to assist your Reiki practice when working with dogs.

Reiki's Uses

Reiki maintains health, heals illnesses and injuries on all levels, and can ease the transition between life and death. It's important to realize that "healing" doesn't necessarily mean physical cure; healing could mean a spiritual rebalancing before a being passes on. Since Reiki is spiritual energy and exists both throughout and beyond the physical realm, you can use Reiki by putting hands directly on the body, or without physical contact.

TRY THIS

Traditional Reiki Exercise: The Joshin Kokyu Ho

(*The Reiki Sourcebook*, pp. 258–59)

Place your hands in your lap, palms facing upward, and close your eyes. Set your intent to be open to receive whatever you need most for healing. With each inhale, feel the energy moving in through your nose, filling your body with energy, all the way down to your hara (the energy center located two or three finger widths below your navel). As you breathe out, see this energy expanding outward, through your skin, into your aura, into the room, and out into the universe. Repeat this visualization as you breathe in and out.

Depending on your comfort level, practice this exercise for anywhere from a few minutes up to a half-hour. In the beginning, you might feel dizzy as you practice building up the energy in your hara. Just take it slow and build up gradually. This exercise is an excellent way to visualize your roots going deeper into the earth. This will serve you well as you do Reiki work with animals. It will help you remain stable, no matter what situation the animal is facing.

Remember that all things consist of energy, so this balancing and harmonizing potential exists for water, food, plants, and even the energy of rooms and other objects. Reiki is not only a way to heal others; it's also a way to bring healing and harmony to your own life every day, supporting all life's situations, both the ups and the downs. And in fact, when we learn to do this for ourselves, it becomes easier then to help our dogs.

Reiki for Self-Healing

Reiki runs much deeper than can be physically observed and understood; it encompasses the emotional, mental, and spiritual aspects of individuals, too. Humans connect more deeply to Reiki by spending time in nature, particularly with animals such as dogs, who inherently and instinctively live closer to nature's way.

Dogs don't need a "system" to heal—as such they don't technically "practice Reiki"; they just naturally live in the flow of the energy, able to utilize its power almost effortlessly. So when we begin to explore this flow of energy our dogs will be there to guide us along the way. By using our heart's compassionate intention, along with some of the simple meditative techniques in this book, we can harness healing energy and create a space that can support dogs who need and want healing. In essence, we can assist them in a return to balance and

TRY THIS
Meditative Exercise with the Five Precepts

For today only:

- Do not anger
- Do not worry
- Be humble
- Be honest in your work
- Be compassionate to yourself and others

Sit quietly with palms resting on the lap or in *gassho* (palms together in front of your throat, a few inches from your body, fingertips facing upward). Recite each precept when you first wake up and right before you go to sleep at night. This exercise cultivates mindfulness of the precepts. Mikao Usui believed the precepts were foundational to one's spiritual development. Practicing the precepts helps to bring balance to your daily life.

harmony through the system of Reiki, which offers practical steps to help us utilize our healing gifts.

The practice of Reiki is not just about connecting with the language of nature and using compassionate intention to support your dog; it's about discovering your true nature, your true essence. Reiki involves more than hoping for good without bad, light without dark, happiness without sadness; it's about understanding that both sides need to be in balance. Without one side, the other could not exist. Only when we remain in balance can we discover true healing and follow nature's way most closely. Learning to embrace both halves of the whole of existence, both sides of the yin and yang, earth as well as heaven, our highest potential as well as our shadow side—this is the way of Reiki.

The foundation of all Reiki healing—the real way you help your dog—is self-practice and meditation. You will need to uncover and explore the areas where you yourself need to heal—and become more open to the flow of energy all around you by completely letting go. As such, although much of this book will focus on using Reiki to work with dogs, I will also be discussing Reiki self-treatment.

The Japanese Energy Centers

According to Japanese philosophy, as taught by Frans and Bronwen Stiene of the International House of Reiki, there are three energy centers in the body: the *hara* (below the navel), which connects you with earth energy; the *middle hara* (found at your heart), which connects you with your human experi-

TRY THIS
Gassho Meditation
(*The Reiki Sourcebook*, p. 253)

Sit in *gassho* (palms together in front of your throat, a few inches from your body, fingertips facing upward), center the mind, and set your intent to begin. Close your eyes and breathe in naturally, focusing on the point where your two middle fingers come together. When your mind wanders, use this physical point to bring yourself back to your focus. Continue for up to 30 minutes.

ence; and the *upper hara* (found in your head), which connects you with heaven energy. (See *The Reiki Sourcebook* for more information about the hara energetic system.)

It's always advisable to build a strong foundation in earth energy first, so that you can remain grounded and stable in all situations. This allows you to be able to provide a space of peace, harmony, and courage no matter what situation an animal may face.

This same advice can be found in one of the Meiji Emperor's *waka* (traditional Japanese poems) which were often used as meditation tools in early Reiki teachings:

> *In a world of storms*
> *Let there be no wavering*
> *Of our human hearts;*
> *Remain as the pine tree*
> *With root sunk deep in stone.*
> —Usui Hikkei

Humans are tactile creatures and, as the energy flows through us, we often feel it more strongly as coming through our hands. In reality, though, Reiki flows through all our energy centers and pathways and is moving throughout our whole body. The traditional techniques and teachings of the Japanese system of Reiki (some of which I share in this book) allow you to deepen your connection to this energy flow. I have included in this book many energy exercises I have found to be of particular assistance when working with dogs. The more you practice with Reiki, the more you will be aware of and feel this energy flow in yourself and all around you.

CHAPTER 4

The Five Precepts: Developing Your Canine Magnetism

Your vision will become clear only when you look into your heart.
Who looks outside, dreams. Who looks inside, awakens.

—Carl Jung

Mikao Usui, the founder of Reiki, wrote the following precepts or rules of conduct to help people live a balanced life.

For today only:

- Do not anger
- Do not worry
- Be humble
- Be honest in your work
- Be compassionate to yourself and others

At its core, Reiki is really about self-healing. Think of the ways we might become unbalanced; this is what leads to a need for healing. The Five Precepts help us remain mindful about staying balanced in our everyday life. When we practice regularly, it becomes easier to stay balanced when we are working with our dogs.

A more balanced energy is also more attractive to a dog, so you may notice that the more you work with the precepts, the easier it is to connect with dogs—not only your own but also others with whom you may come into contact. In this chapter, I'd like to discuss how dogs can help us reflect upon and deepen our connection to the precepts in our lives.

The Importance of Finding Inner Peace: For Today Only, Do Not Anger

For the purposes of this first precept, I'd like to discuss how working with rescued dogs can deepen our understanding and help us go deeper into our own self-healing journey.

As caretakers of rescued dogs, we may find that dealing with the aftereffects of a life of poor treatment is indeed a challenge. In addition, as we develop our connections with rescued dogs through our Reiki treatments, we might begin to feel more protective of them. As we sit with them and offer healing, we may also have to closely observe the suffering and post-traumatic stress that they may be experiencing. In so doing, we might begin to develop a deep intuitive understanding of all the past negative experiences that the dogs have gone through. This is not an easy thing to observe and accept from a peaceful place.

We might begin to feel ourselves becoming very angry about how the dog was treated, what he or she had to go through, and so on. This anger at the dog's past can spiral into anger about the world as a whole—and anger about human-ity's treatment of dogs in general. Pretty soon we might find ourselves encompassed in a bubble of anger. Our focus be-comes anger, so our energy moves in that direction. This anger will merely distract us from our primary goal, which is to help the dog. In addition, if we are angry, the dog will sense that and may not want to connect with us. Energetically, anger is heavy, dark, and restrictive; it doesn't leave much room for the light of healing to shine through.

It's good to admit the anger we may feel in ourselves and reflect upon it. In our reflections, we might begin to realize that holding a focus on anger within our own energy detracts from our ability to create a space of healing. Yes, there has been suffering. Yes, the dog has many hurdles to jump over in order to be healed. Yes, it is a difficult thing to move beyond such a difficult past. But most importantly, we must recognize that despite all this, the dog really wants to heal. He or she wants to let go and move beyond the past into a bright and loving future. If we, too, can let go of our anger, we can ex-pand our perception of the situation to see that where there is hope, there is light and healing possibility.

Instead of focusing on the anger, if we can focus instead on our desire to help the dog, the anger can begin to be miti-gated by our compassion. The healing potential of a happy future for the dog becomes real to us. Our focus can then shift into the positive. When we can let go of anger, it can also help us to see the dog with our heart instead of our eyes. If we can see deeper into the very essence and spirit of the dog—see that bright star just waiting to shine—it will be easier to work through any difficulties we might face, with patience and calm. Instead of being narrow and limited within the dark emotion of anger, our perception becomes as expansive as the universe within the light of compassion and healing possibility.

In letting go of anger, we can begin to see beyond the outer layers of suffering and into the inner nature and potential of the dog. Seeing the deeper spirit of a wounded animal—realizing how perfect the inner spirit of the dog is, even in this moment where healing is needed—brings a strong sense of peace within ourselves. It renews our sense of purpose in supporting the dog and strengthens our compassionate connection with them. When we approach our rescued dog with this kind of faith in healing possibility, we radiate an inner peace. In turn, we will find an enthusiastic and willing Reiki partner—a dog who cannot wait to connect to us and relax into the Reiki space of peace and possibility.

The Importance of Grounding: Just for Today, Do Not Worry

I live near Muir Woods, an incredible national monument of old-growth redwood forest, with trees as tall as 200 feet or more reaching 500 to 1,200 years of age. It is an incredible place to visit. The energy emanating from the trees is palpable; it is just so strong. Walking through this forest, I marvel at how these trees can stand up so straight and tall for so long without falling, without being affected by the changing of the seasons, the coming and going of the years and decades. Our short lives as humans and animals seem so small and insignificant in comparison. The trees reach up to the sky, but I notice they also must maintain a healthy root system to stay stable within the earth.

Some students have asked me, "How do I protect myself from taking on bad energy from my dog's disease?" or "How do I guard myself from the emotions of the past of a dog at the shelter?" For me, the trees in Muir Woods show us the way. The best answer I can give is: We must learn to ground ourselves.

It is natural, of course, to feel emotional about working with dogs with health problems because we care about them. But when we get knocked over by those emotions, this can become a problem as we are not able to hold a space of healing to support the dog. I think of TV weather reports I've watched during a hurricane, where the video footage shows a random tree flying by during high-force winds. We don't want to end up like that uprooted tree, overcome by emotions, literally "blown away" in our pursuit of helping others. In reality, we can't help our dogs if we can't stay stable and grounded. We want to remain like the tall and strong redwood trees—sure and balanced through it all.

When we inquire into the emotions that underlie our wanting to protect ourselves during a Reiki treatment, we will usually see that the primary emotion is fear—fear of taking on something that is not ours, fear of connecting with something disturbing or difficult in the animal, fear of facing our own issues about particular healing situations our dogs face, and so on. The goal of Reiki is to connect—to become one with our dog. How can we do this if we are coming from a place of fear?

We must return to the second Reiki precept: Just for to-day, do not worry. If we truly let go of fear, we enter a space of pure compassion, where we are not afraid of picking up something negative; in fact, we might find ourselves in such a loving space we would willingly take on every health issue if it would mean healing for our dogs. Think of a mother's love for her child—there is nothing that she would not do for him or her, even giving her own life. Such compassion is a beautiful thing, and something that Reiki can help us to learn to cultivate in all our relationships, with humans and animals. When we connect in the space of Reiki, we enter a place full of perfect balance and harmony. Yes, perhaps there are issues that we ourselves need to work on—and the animals may mirror these for us. Maybe we feel especially upset, for example, when an animal has a past abuse issue. Maybe we, too, have dealt with that issue in the past but haven't worked through it completely. Maybe sitting with our dog as he or she is dying brings up our own mortality feelings and concerns. It might not feel very comfortable for us. Our dogs have a way of pointing us to our own healing concerns and helping us work through those concerns, even as they make their own journeys through this life.

Energetically, fear is small, closed, and restrictive. Like a cage, it separates us from the ones we love. But by sitting with our dogs, contemplating our fears, and slowly learning to let go of them, we open more fully to the present moment however it looks, and it becomes easier to walk this road of healing.

The power of the earth is strong, protective, deep, and reliable. In connecting with the earth regularly, we can begin to realize that it is not something separate from us. It is a power that is part of who we are, and thus always accessible to us. If we can practice opening up to earth energy, we can develop our energetic foundation so that even when we experience self-healing challenges, or sit with our dogs during difficult times, it becomes easier to access this inner strength, let go of fear, and find our balance. It is in a balanced state that we can expand more easily to access our highest compassion. Our dogs will come forward eagerly to share this strong and stable space of healing with us.

The Importance of Opening to Animal Wisdom: Be Humble

I have found that one of the most helpful ways to win over my canine clients is to be mindful of the way I approach the dog. Coming from a place of humility when I am with them is key; it brings us back to the third precept, "Be humble." Yes, I am human. Yes, perhaps I know a little bit about the healing issues my dogs are facing. But in reality, I can only ever know a small piece of the bigger puzzle that represents the whole picture—the life, destiny, purpose, and spirit of the dog. When I am working with Reiki, I might connect very deeply to the dog and begin to understand something about the healing process. I know, though, that it is the dog who is healing himself; I am merely supporting the process as best as I can.

If I go into a treatment thinking, "I know what is wrong, and I'm here to heal this dog," this often results in a dog who is very resistant or unwilling to connect with Reiki. Energetically, it can feel like they are being "pushed," and they might not like it.

On the other hand, if my energy communicates that "I am here to hold a space of healing. I invite you to connect with me in this space for whatever you need at this moment," the vibration is very different. It is then up to the dog to connect and come forward, for whatever they are open to receive. It honors their wisdom and the fact that this healing journey belongs to them, not to us.

Many dogs will literally come forward and "ask" for Reiki when we approach them in this humble way. So in a very important way, humility builds trust in the Reiki relationship. And again, this goes back again to the idea that the dogs are our teachers, not just our Reiki clients.

Coming from a humble place has a way of turning the tables—in a good way. As we deepen our connections with the dog through Reiki, we might find that our lives are forever changed for the better and our hearts are opening more than we had ever thought possible. In working through the healing journey of our dog, we may also learn about ourselves. In so doing, we might actually find that we are better people for it and one day realize that it is we who were healed by our dogs. I am humbled by a dog's capacity to heal and forgive, to let go of the past, and to move forward into a new future with courage, joy, and selfless devotion. If only we could learn to live our lives as dogs live theirs.

The Importance of Being True to Yourself: Be Honest in Your Work

For me, dogs are great examples of being true to yourself. They are who they are, purely and simply, without apology and without judgment. They make it look easy, don't they? We humans seem to find it so difficult to follow our hearts, to be true to our life's purpose, to let go of our worries and other complications and just "be." We get caught up in so many of life's daily responsibilities, forgetting to be present, to feel our inner truth, and have the courage to follow our hearts. It reminds me of the old Zen proverb: "Before enlightenment, chop wood, carry water. After enlightenment, chop wood, carry water."

Being true and open and honest should not be something that we only find for ourselves on a rare occasion in our lives. We must remember to be open and present and in a space of compassion all the time, even when doing the menial tasks of daily life. How much easier it would be to enjoy each precious and fragile moment on this earth, if we did this. This is the lesson our dogs teach us: how to enjoy each moment fully. Think of your dog when he or she is playing, napping, eating, or taking a walk. You can see how pure and fully open they are to each moment. It is a beautiful thing.

As we go through our days, how often do we really take a look at our life, contemplate it, and ask ourselves, What is my life's work? And do we practice this work each and every day? If we look deeply beneath the surface of things, and if we are really honest with ourselves, the only true "work" we must practice always is and must only ever be the work of our deepest soul.

How can we get in touch with this deeper part of ourselves on a daily basis? Our dogs can help us. Being who they are in their own skin, they find it easier to be more fully present each and every moment. So when we share time with them, they can help bring us into their space of being. When we support our dogs, when we are helping them heal, nurturing them physically and emotionally, providing exercise, food,

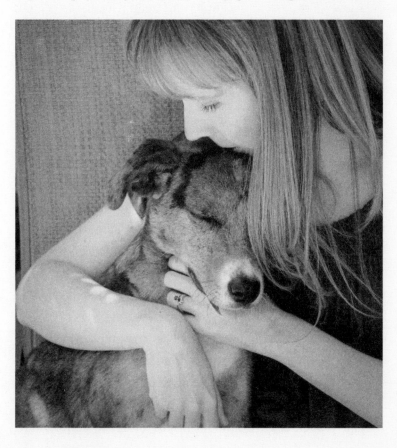

and attention, we are also learning about compassion and openness and honesty.

We can realize that it is in this daily life with our dogs, where we devote ourselves openly to our simple tasks of caring for them, that we are more easily able to uncover our heart's true calling. In helping our dogs to heal and live life surrounded in love, we might effortlessly find ourselves expanded in a place of compassion where we, too, can be truly honest in our soul's work. And our dogs will love us for it!

The Importance of Living with Kindness: Be Compassionate to Yourself and Others

Helping a dog is, of course, a compassionate action, which I believe has a ripple effect out into the world, both physically and spiritually. In one way, you are modeling how to be self-compassionate. The gentleness and kindness that is so easy for you to show your dog is something you might try practicing with yourself. Although animal caretaking comes very naturally for many of us, being loving and kind to ourselves might be a bit more difficult. So practicing this loving kindness with our dogs can help us get better at our own practice of self-love.

The circle of kindness expands ever farther. By working with dogs in our lives, we are not only helping each individual dog in our care but also, by being a model for others in this work, we are helping to pave the way toward a more compassionate planet. Our work might inspire others to do the same.

If each of us does his or her small part for the dogs in our lives, imagine how all those little acts of compassion can build up and grow all around the world. How wonderful to know that we are not alone, and there are so many others helping dogs everywhere!

Spiritually, by helping the dogs you love, it is as if you are placing a loving embrace around all the dogs in the world who don't have anyone to love them. We are all connected, and every little act of kindness expands out into the universe in a very healing way. So knowing this, be kind and gentle to yourself. You may not be able to save every dog, but you can make a difference in your own life for the dogs who may cross your path.

And this kindness and love will expand beyond what your physical eyes can see, in heart-healing ways, all across the planet. In following your heart for the dogs in need, you will develop the compassionate spirit within you and nurture the compassionate spirit on this planet. With practice, you will begin to see that dogs can actually sense this space of light within you and are drawn to connect with you in that space.

PART II

ADAPTING REIKI TREATMENTS FOR DOGS

Your work is to discover your world
and then with all your heart give yourself to it.

—The Buddha

CHAPTER 5

Overview of Canine Reiki Basics

Follow your bliss and don't be afraid, and doors will open where you didn't know they were going to be.
—Joseph Campbell

As you set out on this journey to help the dogs you care for so deeply, it's good to keep in mind that these animals—big or small, well-known to you or strangers, affectionate or aloof— will all be your teachers in one way or another. That's because when it comes to working with Reiki healing energy and learning to speak the subtle language of connection with all things, dogs are truly masters. It takes practice to listen, to connect, to feel, and to understand. It takes time and patience to begin to uncover the profound quality of the energy you are offering. But for dogs, this is second nature. They will not only be your helpers; they will be your leaders on the journey.

Dogs as Teachers of Energy

In many ways, dogs and humans are very similar spiritual beings. We all experience the ebb and flow of our individual lives. We all have physical, mental, emotional, and spiritual levels. We all have Reiki as our essence.

But there are also many spiritual differences between animals and humans, and it is essential to consider these differences when doing Reiki work with dogs. You must adapt the Reiki treatment to suit the awareness, sensitivities, wisdom, and experience of the dogs you are with if you are to gain their trust and acceptance.

Dogs are more "tuned in" to the energetic realm, and their physical bodies actually help them to be acutely aware of their environment and the beings therein. They are highly

TRY THIS
Exercise to Connect with the Energetic Realm in a Physical Way

Little field trips to sit with the ocean and a tree (see pages 54 and 57) are great ways to connect more deeply with nature and the energetic rhythms that underpin our existence, whether we are aware of it or not. Energy has its own language; in learning Reiki, we are learning to speak this language a little bit at a time. Sitting with the animals in a healing energetic space is a way of connecting and communicating with energy instead of with verbal language: the ebbs and flows, pushes and pulls, and ups and downs in the flow—these are simply the words and phrases of an energetic conversation. The ocean mimics the energy of a Reiki treatment, however, in a very strong physical way, and so is a great place to begin learning to "speak energy." Trees are deeply connected to the earth and the sky, and their quiet, stationary existence can teach us much about being still and learning go deeper within ourselves and listen to our hearts. Indeed, the ocean and trees show us a great deal about energy: movement that resides within stillness, and the stillness that resides within movement.

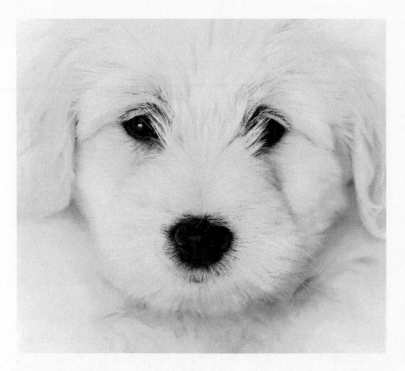

tuned into our physical presence as well, and our behavior, physical movement, and posture during treatment can affect their willingness to accept the energy. To respect their physical sensitivities, we must speak quietly and behave calmly; avoid forcing physical contact with hands-on Reiki (in other words, being willing to maintain the physical distance the animal chooses); avoid dominant physical positions; and maintain respectful and nonconfrontational eye contact (or sometimes avoid eye contact all together).

Dogs have more highly developed intuition than humans do. They sense what we are thinking, feeling, and saying; they can "figure us out"—sometimes even before we've figured ourselves out! The odds of a dog being willing to connect with us

TRY THIS
The Ocean

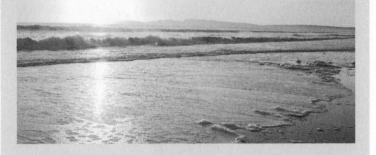

Go to the ocean for a few hours. Sit in the sand near the water, make yourself comfortable, let go of your daily concerns, and just be with the waves. Tune into your five senses: What does the ocean look like? See its movement, shapes, and colors. How does it sound? Listen to it crashing and splashing. What does it smell like? Allow yourself to breathe in the ocean scent deeply and slowly. What might it taste like? (Perhaps you have a memory of a surfing wipeout from the past, or maybe you have tried seaweed at a Japanese restaurant.) How would it feel to be in the waves? (Again, you can draw upon memories of wading in the waves.) Let your memories and senses run wild for a time. After a while you will notice that your thoughts lessen, and you begin to relax and feel the ocean on a deeper level. Time may seem to stand still, and you may feel as if you can stay where you are indefinitely, you are so relaxed and at peace. Notice the ebbs and flows of the wave sets as they come in and out. Notice the tide as it moves up or down the beach. Let the comforting sound, movement, and repetition of the waves carry you away, mentally and spiritually. Begin to feel your connection with the ocean—how the movement inside your own body (pulse, heartbeat, blood circulation, breathing) might echo the movement of the ocean. Notice the stillness that resides deep within the strong motion that is the ocean.

for a Reiki treatment grows when we have positive thoughts, see the dog as fully healed and perfectly in balance, and remain mentally tranquil and open. Conversely, if we focus on the problems and health issues the dogs are displaying, our thoughts may distress them or add to the burden they already carry in dealing with whatever health crisis exists. As Reiki practitioners, it is our job to hold a space of lightness and peace in our minds. In this space, the dog is more likely to relax and open to an energetic connection.

Dogs do not experience the conflicted and complicated emotions humans do. This is one of the reasons we can learn valuable life lessons through observing and supporting a dog's healing journey. By connecting with a calm emotional state inside yourself before you approach any dog for Reiki, you improve the chances of the dog being open to the healing work you are offering. You can't fool dogs by pretending to be calm on the outside while being upset on the inside. They will sense the emotional disconnect, may decide they can't trust you, and probably won't participate in Reiki treatments with you. If you're feeling in any way unbalanced, it's better to wait until a time when you feel calm to offer a Reiki treatment to your dog.

Dogs are closer to spirit on a daily basis than humans are. This is especially apparent when you connect with them during the dying process. Their understanding, acceptance, and surrender throughout the process offer lessons for us humans. Being open to the spiritual process of healing, in both life and death, without expectations, can help us become more receptive to these lessons and gain spiritual wisdom from dogs along the way. Offering Reiki to dogs as they transition fully into spirit form may be some of the most profound energetic experiences you will ever have.

Taking into consideration these fundamental differences between humans and animals in the context of a Reiki treatment, I have developed a core, guiding philosophy—an ethical code—for working with animals and Reiki. I will go into more detail in the next few chapters, but my philosophy is brief and to the point: Let the animals lead the way in Reiki treatments.

In the following chapters, I will guide you through the specific steps every Reiki student or practitioner must know in order to facilitate effective Reiki treatments with any dog. We will start by learning my five golden rules of animal acceptance, which are absolutely critical to the success of any canine Reiki encounter.

I will share with you real-life lessons, tips, and strategies you can use energetically to heal the dogs you love—whether you volunteer in shelters, rehabilitate foster dogs, bond with family pets, or simply want to assist your own beloved dog in making his or her transition to the spiritual realm.

And finally, I will highlight some very important lessons you can expect to learn from the dogs with whom you do energetic healing work. As much as we may wish to rescue dogs, what Reiki practitioners soon find is that the dogs actually rescue us as well—they enrich our lives and make us better people by teaching us profound lessons in courage, forgiveness, hope, and more.

I look forward to joining you on this journey toward spiritual awareness, healing, and a deepened interspecies connection.

TRY THIS
The Tree

Find a big, strong healthy tree in your yard or local area that you can visit quietly, without being disturbed. Sit in the *gassho* meditation posture at the base of the tree (palms together at heart level). Set your intention that you are open to receive whatever you need most at this very moment. Ask the tree to assist you in this.

With your feet about shoulder's width apart, stand close to the tree and place your hands lightly on the trunk. Breathe in and out, with your eyes open in soft focus. Allow your senses to open to all the sounds and smells around you. Imagine the roots of the tree beneath you. Feel the solidity and strength of the tree trunk beneath your hands. Smell the aroma of the tree. See the patterns of the bark and the design of the branches stretching up into the sky above you. Listen to the leaves as they blow in the breeze. Imagine you can breathe in the earth energy beneath you, up through the soles of your feet, and breathe out the crown of your head into the expansiveness of the sky above. Imagine your feet are the tree's roots, your body is the tree's trunk, your head and arms are the tree's branches. Feel yourself 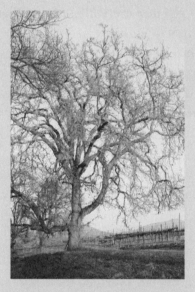 connecting to the energy of the tree, and more than that, becoming one with it. How does it feel to be this tree? Notice the energetic movement that resides deep within the stillness that is the tree. Just stand and be with the tree in this energy of earth and sky for 30 minutes or more.

CHAPTER 6

A Typical Canine Reiki Treatment

Love the animals, love the plants, love everything.
If you love everything, you will perceive the divine
mystery in things.
Once you perceive it, you will begin to comprehend it
better every day.
And you will come at last to love the whole world with
an all-embracing love.

    —Fyodor Dostoyevsky

To build a complete holistic program for your dog's health and wellness, it's important to find a veterinarian that you trust, a nutritious wholefood diet, a training program that is gentle and positive, and of course, a variety of complementary therapies, such as Reiki, for any healing challenges your dog may encounter. Together, these key ingredients will allow your dog to find balance and harmony on all levels.

In my opinion, Reiki is a wonderful complement (and the best supplement) to whatever holistic program you choose for your dog. Reiki can support your dog through all stages of his life, from puppyhood to aging senior. You can offer Reiki to all the animals in your household together—it's a great way to spend healing family time. Reiki can also support relaxation and relieve stress in dogs of all energy levels and temperaments. Reiki can be effective in any environment, from a loving home to an overcrowded and underfunded shelter. Reiki always brings peace and harmony. There is no situation (physical, emotional, or spiritual) that it cannot support.

When offering Reiki to dogs, it's good to set aside 30 to 60 minutes of uninterrupted time, if possible. Find a comfortable position from which to do the treatment. Make sure your spine is straight and shoulders, arms, and legs are relaxed so that the energy can flow easily through you. Sit in meditation and think of "holding the space" for healing for the dog for that length of time. Try not to worry about what the dog is or is not doing, where they are, whether they are sleeping or lying down, and so on. This mental chatter interferes with

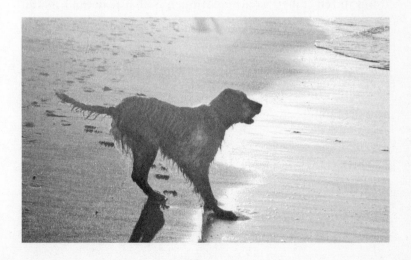

our ability to let go into the energetic space. The more we can just open to the energy, the more stable and strong a healing environment we create for the dog.

I usually begin with three or four Reiki treatments on consecutive days. Healing treatments are cumulative: If you can do them close together, it's likely that you will see positive results in just a few days. After these initial treatments, I wait and see how the dog is doing to determine how often to follow up. When the dog seems to need support again, that's the time for more Reiki. It might be once or twice a month or once or twice a week; it depends on the dog and the health challenge.

When dogs accept a Reiki treatment, typically there are several things you might see happen. For example, dogs show lots of movement to and from the person during treatment. I call this the "ebb and flow" of a treatment. They also will typically greet us at the beginning of a treatment and "say thank you" at the end of the treatment. The most important thing to remember, as a practitioner, is that it doesn't matter whether or not there is physical contact: The dog will be able to connect with the healing energy even from a distance. Often you will also observe signs of relaxation in the dog, such as yawns, sighs, sitting or lying down, and perhaps even sleep and dreaming.

Using Your Hands in a Reiki Treatment

Many dogs enjoy hands-on Reiki treatments, and they will show you this by approaching you and placing their bodies under your hands. It is wonderful when an animal chooses to receive hands-on treatment. There are a few things to remember when using hands-on contact during Reiki.

- **Create a soft, mental focus.** Try not to focus your thoughts on your hands, even if you are touching the dog. Don't visualize the energy as flowing out your palms and into the dog's body. Instead, imagine that Reiki is flowing through your entire body, mind, and spirit, encompassing the space all around you. This will create a softer mental vibration as you offer Reiki to your dog.

- **Use light, gentle touch.** Reiki is not massage and does not require any pressure. Your hands may be motionless or you may lightly pet the dog (sometimes this is comforting for the dog), or you might plant one hand on the dog while the other hand slowly pets him or her. Watch the dog's body language to see how they feel most comfortable and relaxed.

- **Relax your fingers.** Don't worry about things like the position of your fingers and palms. Just relax your hands lightly on the body of the animal. Your palm may be flat against the dog, or only your fingertips and edge of palm may be touching the animal, with your hand lightly cupped.

- **Movement is not needed unless your dog wishes it.** If your dog is comfortable, there is no need to move your hands during treatment; you can keep them in one position that feels good to your dog. However, your dog's body language may show you that it's time to move your hands (your dog may change positions under your hands or give you a meaningful look and then relax again once you move your hands.) Be open and flexible about what makes your dog the most relaxed and the most comfortable. This is exactly the right way to "be" with your hands.

- **Follow your intuition.** As the treatment progresses, you may notice yourself changing your hand positions, either moving closer to the animal (for example, going from a lightly cupped hand to a flat hand) or farther away from the animal (for example, removing physical contact by placing your hands a few inches above the dog's body.) As long as the dog is remaining relaxed and happy, you can know that you are doing the "right" hand positions.

Treatment Guidelines

- Spend a few moments connecting to the energy through breathing or meditation.
- Greet the dog.
- Ask permission/set intention.
- Sit in the space of energy for 30 to 60 minute. Place yourself 5 to 10 feet away from the dog. Only offer hands-on Reiki if the dog moves close to you or into your hands. Your eyes might be open or closed. Rest your hands on your lap, palms up or palms down, or keep them in *gassho* (palms together in front of your heart). Bring yourself back to focus when needed by repeating the breathing/meditation exercises.

- Thank the dog for his openness to connecting. Set your intention to finish.

The following is an example of a Reiki session I had with one dog, Bruce.

In photo 1, I have my hands in *gassho* and am asking permission/setting my intention to offer Reiki for Bruce, for whatever he is open to receive, or nothing at all. I always like to remind dogs each time I connect with them that it is totally up to them, totally their choice to take part or not.

In photo 2, Bruce senses the Reiki energy and turns around to connect with me through eye contact. In essence, he is saying "yes" to the treatment.

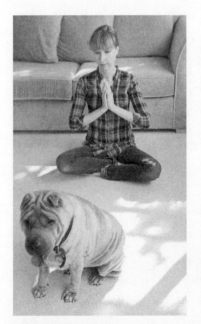 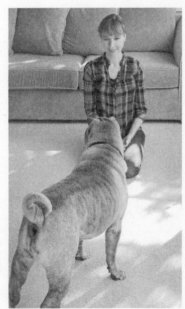

Photo 1 (left): Kathleen asking for permission to offer Reiki.
Photo 2 (right): Bruce senses the Reiki energy.

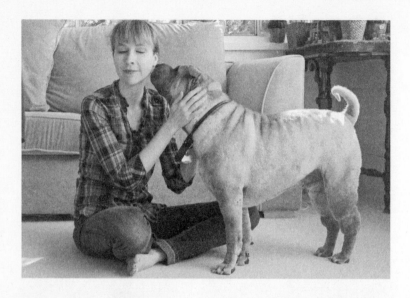

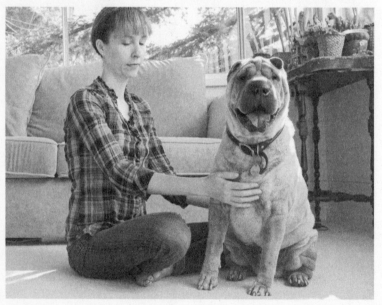

Photo 3 (top): Bruce accepts the offer of Reiki.

Photo 4 (bottom): Bruce settles near Kathleen for the treatment.

In photo 3, Bruce is coming close to greet me and engage with me in the Reiki connection. This is a wonderful example of the gratitude we often see animals display when they feel the energy we offer.

In photo 4, Bruce decides to settle close by me, and I respond by placing my hands on him where they seem to intuitively go. I can tell he accepts these hand positions because he stays put and does not move away.

In photo 5, Bruce decides to move again and lie down next to me. Rather than moving toward him, I simply place

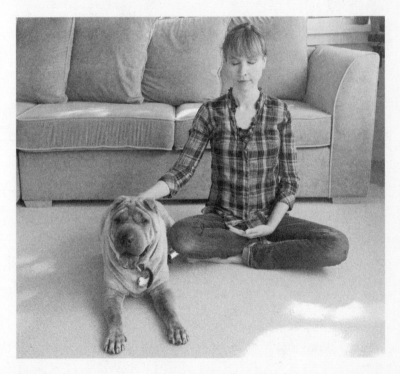

Photo 5: It's best to always keep a physical position that encourages relaxation.

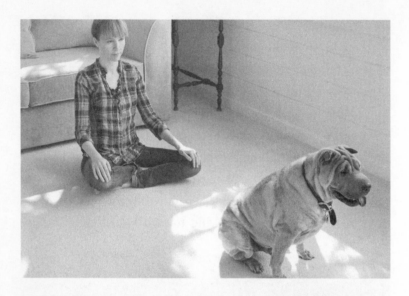

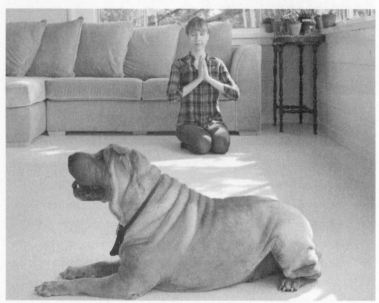

Photo 6 (top): After several minutes, Bruce moves away.

Photo 7 (bottom): Bruce walks even farther away during treatment.

my hands in a relaxed manner, one hand in my lap and one on Bruce. It's best to always keep a physical position that encourages relaxation, so that we do not become distracted because we feel uncomfortable. Also, we don't need to be directly facing the dog when we are treating them—they might be in front of us, to the side, or even directly behind us. Just relax into the meditation and try to resist the urge to keep shifting your position to be facing the dog.

In photo 6, after several minutes, Bruce moves away from me, facing in the opposite direction. I choose to rest my hands where they feel comfortable: You can do this palms up or palms down on your lap. Try to relax and feel the connection with your whole being, rather than focusing on your hands.

In photo 7, Bruce walks even farther away and lies down to relax at a distance from me. Again, it's important to relax and accept your dog's movement during treatment. I choose to focus on breathing so, without coming closer, I shift my position and move into a *gassho* pose with my hands.

In photo 8, after several more minutes, Bruce comes forward again and gives me strong eye contact. I can feel the connection with him

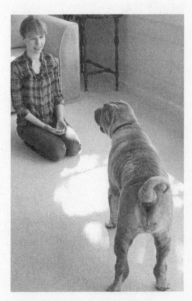

Photo 8: Bruce approaches Kathleen and establishes strong eye contact.

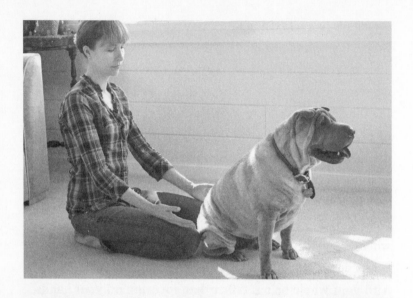

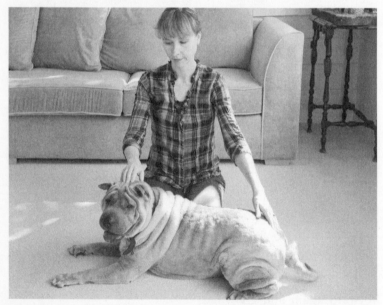

Photo 9 (top): Remember to breathe and allow the connection to unfold naturally.

Photo 10 (bottom): Bruce settles directly in front of Kathleen.

very strongly even at a distance. I stay relaxed and quietly tell him what a good boy he is.

In photo 9, Bruce turns around and presents his hind end at close quarters. I can relax my hands and just continue to feel the connection of the energy with my entire being. I remember to just breathe and allow the connection to unfold naturally.

In photo 10, Bruce finally settles again directly in front of me. Intuitively, my hands are drawn to his head and tail. He relaxes into the position, and I can feel a strong sense of connection and harmony between us.

In photo 11, Bruce shows me he is finished with the treatment by becoming more active and alert and licking my hands as if to say, "Thanks."

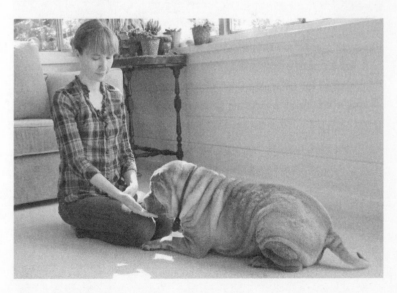

Photo 11: Bruce becomes more active and alert, indicating that the treatment is finished.

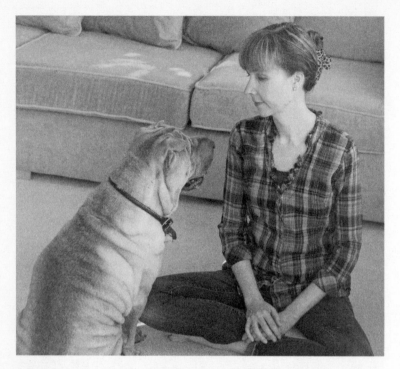

Photo 12: It is common to feel that a deep Reiki bond has been created between you and your dog by the end of the treatment.

After the treatment, in photo 12, Bruce comes forward so that he can look right at me. It is common to feel that a deep Reiki bond has been created between you and your dog by the end of the treatment. Some dogs show this with eye contact or other physical contact (like a paw on the arm, a lick on the face, or little nudge from the nose). There can be a deep feeling of trust and connection even after just a short period of time, when your dog has truly opened to healing within the Reiki space.

PART III

Building the Bridge of Healing Possibility

The morning sun

Rises so splendidly

Into the sky;

Oh, that we could attain

Such a clear reviving soul!

—*Waka* by Meiji Emperor,
translated by Professor Harold Wright

CHAPTER 7

Preparing to Offer Reiki

*The most precious gift we can offer others is our
presence.*
*When mindfulness embraces those we love, they will
bloom like flowers.*
—Thich Nhat Hanh

For some of you reading this book, this may be the first time
you've tried working with energy. You may find yourself open
to trying something new because you have found that all
other allopathic methods have run their course. The whole
concept of "connecting and healing with energy" may seem
very foreign to you. This is just fine. Your animal has brought
you to this place, and he or she will guide you along as you
move farther. Remember the quote by Zen master Shunryu
Suzuki: "In the beginner's mind there are many possibilities,
but in the expert's there are few." Your newness to energy
work, along with your heartfelt wish to help your animal, is
the perfect setup for a powerful healing space. So sit back,
relax, and be open to whatever comes to you.

Heal Yourself First

I first learned Reiki as a tool for self-healing. I had struggled with anxiety and worry my whole life and was ready to try anything to get better. As I began working with Reiki energy, I

TRY THIS
The Healing Bridge Meditation
(special thanks to Tosha Silver for the earth and sky imagery)

Close your eyes and take a deep breath. Let it out slowly. Take another deep breath. Let it out slowly. Imagine that all of your stresses from the day release from you with each exhale. Breathe in. Exhale slowly. Allow yourself to let go of all your concerns and just be aware of your breath.

Imagine there are roots coming down from the base of your spine. These roots stretch far down into the earth, grounding you. Feel yourself stable, grounded, part of the earth, just as if you were a beautiful tree. Imagine that the grounding energy of the earth can flow up these roots into your heart center, giving you stability and peace.

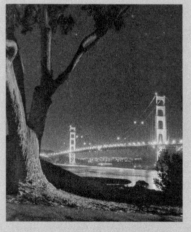

Now imagine that the expansive, creative energy of the sky is flowing down into your crown chakra. It is a beautiful rain of light, healing, and goodness. It flows from your crown, into your heart chakra, and out through your hands. It mingles with the energy of the earth to give you a perfect blend of the physical and the divine within you. You can feel the energy of the earth and sky flowing within your whole being. Earth and sky energy would sit each day and offer myself healing energy. Although I was a complete beginner, I somehow knew that only by becoming familiar with the energy, working with it and "sitting" with it every day, could healing begin to happen inside myself.

come in, mix together, and go out until you feel a beautiful white column of light spreading within your whole being.

Now bring to your mind an animal who has motivated you to be here today to learn Reiki. See the animal here with you right now. I'd like you to imagine you can build a bridge of healing light, of healing earth and sky energy, to your animal. See this bridge extending out from your heart to the heart of your animal. This bridge represents an offering of healing light, of Reiki. It represents the possibility of healing on whatever level is needed most by your animal and a chance to find balance, peace, and harmony. Your animal has a choice now in how, or whether, to accept your offering. He or she may stay on the other side, choose to step a paw or hoof or claw or two on the bridge, meet you halfway, or perhaps walk all the way across to you.

Allow yourself to let go of your expectations about what the animal should do, and just focus on offering the healing light from your heart to your animal's heart, embracing their freedom of choice. Imagine what might happen with the bridge of light and your animal's decision.

After several minutes, thank your animal for his openness to healing possibilities, and for the lessons he has yet to teach you in healing. Slowly bring your energy bridge back to yourself. Bring all your energy back, easily and completely. Feel your energy returning to you, feel your breath returning to you. Feel yourself again bathed in the white column of light connecting you to the power of the earth and the expansiveness of the sky.

When you are ready, take a nice, deep cleansing breath and slowly come back and open your eyes, feeling refreshed and at peace.

As much as I've always loved animals throughout my life, initially it didn't occur to me to offer them Reiki. So when my dog began to crawl onto my feet every time I offered myself Reiki, it was a bit confusing. Finally, it dawned on me that he was feeling the energy, enjoying it, and clearly—as evidenced by his long sighs, yawns, and deep sleep—using it for his own healing. I hadn't intentionally "offered" healing to him, yet here he was making the most of the energy.

So, strange as it may seem, my understanding of animal Reiki began to unfold at the same time as my own self-practice. Today, self-healing work remains the foundation of all my animal Reiki work.

What Exactly Happens When You Give a Reiki Treatment to Your Animal?

Giving Reiki is a kind of meditation. You are simply creating an energetic space, and in this space, healing can happen. You allow yourself to get in touch with that fundamental connection you have with others and, indeed, all things in the universe. By simply relaxing, being quiet, breathing, and having a heartfelt intention to help another being, you create a sacred space. In this space, all things are possible. You simply allow the energy to flow in through your body and out toward the animal.

When the energy flows through you, you may feel sensations in your hands, arms, or body such as heat, buzzing, pulsing, deep relaxation, peace, and harmony. You may find your mind becoming very quiet and may feel "far away." Your thoughts and mental activity may begin to dissipate for a time. With regular practice, you will begin to feel the energetic ebbs and flows within your physical and emotional being (ups and downs in the flow of the energy). The more you can relax your physical and mental self during the treatment and just open to the process, the easier it will be to sense the energy. Sensing the energy takes regular practice; being with animals daily as you practice, observing and listening to them, can speed up your energy "learning curve."

You could say that we Reiki practitioners use our intention and focus to create a sort of "healing bridge." The bridge is built upon the foundation of our personal Reiki meditation and treatment practice, energetic experience, purity of intention, and the trust we create with the animals. The bridge itself consists of the purity of balance, harmony, and connection or "oneness" that is the essence of Reiki, the energetic "stuff" that makes up everything in the universe.

The question always is, What will an animal do when presented with the bridge? It's like the old saying, "You can lead a horse to water, but you cannot make him drink." You cannot force a Reiki healing treatment upon anyone; you simply build the bridge. The animal is then presented with a healing possibility, and what he decides to do with that healing possibility is his own decision. He may come to the edge of the bridge and just put one little paw onto it. He may meet us in the middle. He may walk all the way across the bridge and cuddle into our arms. Or he may turn and walk away.

When the animal chooses to walk this bridge of healing (whether it be tentatively or with great enthusiasm), each step is a miracle of self-healing on the part of the animal, supported by the energetic balance and harmony of the bridge we have created.

Who Is Doing the Healing?

It's important to realize that you offer the energy to facilitate healing; *you* do not actually "heal" the animal. Nor do you control where the energy is going, or indeed whether it is going at all. You cannot decide, "I'm going to send Reiki to this animal's broken leg now," or "I think I should send energy to heal this animal's anxiety." Yes, you may think you know what the animal needs, but in reality, since the animal is completely responsible for his or her own healing process, he or she will decide whether or not to accept the energy you offer. Healing is a uniquely personal experience; it cannot be forced upon another individual.

I remember once offering a treatment to my horse in his pasture. After several minutes of standing very near me, he turned and walked to the other side of the pasture to graze. Usually, this would indicate to me that he was finished with the treatment; however, I still felt a very strong flow of energy within my body. I thought to myself, "Well, I guess he's just wanting energy from farther away today." I continued to stand there and allow the energy to flow to him (or so I thought). After some time, I felt the energy ebb and knew the treatment was over.

I thanked him, turned to leave the pasture, and was surprised by what I saw. The horse in the neighboring pasture, whom I didn't know well and who always kept his distance from me, had come to the very edge of the fence, just behind me, and was sleeping soundly, his eyes closed and head hanging very low. I realized that he was the reason I had felt the energy so strongly after my own horse had gone to the other end of the field. But it didn't really matter what I thought was happening, or where I imagined the energy was going: Because I was open to facilitating the process, some animals in my vicinity were open to accepting the energy, and healing was able to take place.

Because its essence is pure balance and harmony, healing energy will go to support the places that need healing most, restoring balance and harmony. Reiki may address the issues that you thought needed healing, or it may travel somewhere else all together. For example, many times an animal may have a skin condition that stems from stress. This is seen a lot in shelter settings. Or an animal could have an emotional condition that actually stems from a traumatic event in the past. Reiki goes like a magnet to the origin of the issues, whatever they are, without needing the practitioner to know what the problem is. You simply need to set your intent and let the energy "do its thing."

Sometimes you can feel as if you are "sending" the energy to what is needed most, but this is merely illusion. On many occasions, I have gone into a treatment thinking I was healing one thing then ended up watching an amazing transformation and healing on an entirely deeper level—or for a different issue, often one of which I was completely unaware. After having so many experiences like this, I realized that, in fact, even if I think I know what the animal needs and feel as if I am directing the energy to heal something specific, the energy goes where it needs to go, regardless.

That's probably the hardest thing about working with energy: getting out of your ego and allowing it to just flow through you clearly and without judgment or control. That's also why it's important that you set aside time for self-healing every day.

Try to allow 30 minutes each morning after you wake up, or in the evening just before bed, to practice the Five Precepts meditation (page 32) or Joshin Kokyu Ho meditation (page 31). In addition, you will want to begin to connect with your animal on a daily basis. Start with a few minutes and build to a 30 to 60 minute meditation. There are many meditations in this book you can try using. You might start with the Healing Bridge Meditation (page 74).

Because you are the channel through which energy flows, you can actually get in your own way if you are distracted, annoyed, or, even worse, overwhelmed by your own challenges. Or you might be so controlling—focused on healing one particular issue—that you lose touch with your intuitive wisdom and entirely miss the healing that Reiki creates because it occurs in an unexpected area. The more you can work on yourself, the deeper you can go into the energy, and the clearer the flow will be when you offer it to others. It's really about learning to "let go and let Reiki."

CHAPTER 8

Golden Rule No. 1: "Speak Energy" with Your Dog

We are what we think.
All that we are arises with our thoughts.
With our thoughts, we make our world.
   —The Buddha

In offering Reiki to your dog, you are about to engage in a subtle, but profound "conversation." This conversation takes place in a language in which you are most likely not fluent. You may already have a good communication and relationship with your dog, and this will serve as a great foundation from which to start. Don't worry, though—all dogs speak "energy" fluently. And most of them are very patient. If we can simply reach out to them with the right attitude, our dogs can become willing teachers in the language of energy.

   As a beginner in this new language, you want to do your utmost to create a trusting and respectful connection. In the beginning, because you are a new student, you may not be able to sense clearly what is going on energetically. This is why I always recommend to beginners practicing Reiki with a dog to always ask his or her permission.

Because animals are so sensitive to energy and already speak this language so well, it's all about the approach. It's about an attitude of humility and respect. It's about giving the animal choice and control. It's about remembering, "Hey, maybe my animal knows more about this than I do." If you don't ask their permission, many animals will choose to walk away from you, thereby shunning your offer of a healing bridge.

By asking permission of your dog before you begin, you establish a clear dynamic between you that will be strengthened each time you connect energetically. You are letting them know that, when it comes to receiving Reiki, they are in charge and can decide. You may be your dogs' caretaker, the person who does everything for them, from visits to the vet or for other holistic treatments, giving them their pills or remedies, feeding and bathing them, and taking them for walks, play, and exercise—but your dogs will take the lead in their own Reiki healing. It may feel funny at first to set up their leadership in this way, but with practice it will become a habit—one to which your dogs will respond very happily!

When you hold a simple intent inside, asking your dog silently to participate rather than telling him or her, "You need healing now because I have decided that you do," you set up a trust relationship between the two of you. The more your dog trusts that it is his or her own choice to participate, the more open he or she will be to the process. Practice asking permission, then sitting with your dog, observing his or her response, over and over. It will help develop your energetic sensitivity and awareness about what is happening in your Reiki connection and your dog's healing process.

Ways to Ask

It's actually very simple to ask your dog's permission. It's more about your intention than about the way you do the asking or the actual words you use. If you are respectful and mindful in your approach, you really can't do it "wrong."

When you are ready to ask for your dog's permission, you can approach him or her and be physically close as you ask, or you can ask from across the room or yard. In reality, this "asking of permission" is about making a clear inner intention or energetic statement, rather than having an actual verbal exchange (although in some cases, you may find yourself doing both!). Offering the Reiki treatment to your dog will in itself be an energetic conversation, so it's good to begin to practice "speaking" in energetic terms right from the start.

There are a couple of ways you can ask permission. The easiest way is aloud, speaking to them softly, "Would you like some Reiki today?" You can do this, for example, as you enter the room where your dogs are hanging out. Then it's great to greet them peacefully and quietly, keeping your energy calm and relaxed, so that they know it's not playtime; your energy is communicating, "It's quiet time—Reiki time." Because as we humans are used to expressing ourselves verbally to show our intention and purpose, making a verbal statement is also a way to "set your energy" or, in other words, make your inner intention known. Dogs read us very easily. They will under-stand what you are saying, not so much by your words but by your energy.

Once you have become accustomed to asking them aloud, you can practice asking permission by forming the question in your mind, "Would you like some Reiki today?" Simply state that sentence inwardly and watch your dog for a reac-tion. Dogs are also very aware of our inner mental attitudes

TRY THIS
Setting Your Intention, Grounding, and Creating a Healing Space

Sit in a quiet space with your animal where you will not be disturbed. Set your intention with words such as, "I set my intention that I am open to facilitate healing for you (the animal), for whatever you are open to receive, or nothing at all. This treatment is completely in your control, and you are totally respon-sible for your own healing. I will simply create a healing space and offer this to you for the next 30 minutes. During that time, you may receive whatever you are comfortable with receiving, for your highest good."

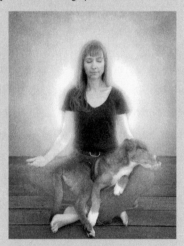

Close your eyes and allow yourself to grow roots down into the earth from the base of your spine. Feel the roots stretching deeply into the earth, grounding you. Feel the energy of the earth flowing up into your heart, grounding you in strength and peace.

and emotions, so when we ask them silently, they do hear us. Think about all the times your dog knew when you were sad or upset and were trying to hide it. And when you were at your happiest and best, your dog shared in that as well. They always know what is going on inside us: We can't hide it from them, even when we try. In the same way, when you set your mental intention to ask permission, they will understand you by your energy.

Now focus for a few minutes on your in-breath. As you inhale, feel your body filling with healing light from the universe. This light flows in as you inhale from the air through your nose and also up from your roots in the earth. Continue to breathe in healing energy from the earth and air as you imagine your body filling as you inhale and becoming a healing column of energy and light.

As you feel your body fill with this beautiful healing energy of perfect harmony of the universe, allow yourself to focus on your out-breath for a few moments. Exhale this column of light out of your body into your aura and into the room you are in. Imagine you can expand the light around you, filling up the space with healing, balance, peace, and harmony.

As you hold this space of healing with your intention for the next several minutes, imagine that your animal can step into and out of the space at his own preference. Try to let go of your expectations about what should happen and simply hold this space of connection and healing for your animal freely and openly. Allow yourself to go deeply into a space of quiet and meditation.

When you are ready, thank your animal for his openness to healing and set your intention to finish. Imagine bringing all your energy back to your body. Bring your awareness back to the here and now. Take a nice deep breath and slowly open your eyes.

Offering Rather Than Giving Reiki

A successful canine Reiki treatment is really about intention and acceptance. To have the best chance of receiving the dog's acceptance of the healing energy you offer, you want to "set your intention" in the most respectful way possible, allowing the animal to take the lead in the treatment.

Practice asking permission, and it will become easier to allow your animal to choose. By the time you reach the intermediate level of Reiki, you will find it easier to let go of your own wishes and desires and begin to understand what it means to "offer" Reiki for your animal rather than "give" Reiki to them.

At this stage in your learning, as you realize this within yourself and relax into the feeling of allowing your animal to lead, you can simply set your intention in a way that is a form of permission. Close your eyes, take a deep, cleansing breath, and as you release your breath, say to yourself, "I set my intention to be an open channel for Reiki healing, for whatever my dog is open to receive, or nothing at all; that is fine, too."

Here you are leaving it up to your dog, without expectation or demanding that he *must* say yes. You are creating an inner focus and intent to be a facilitator not a "dictator" for the healing process. Your dog will feel your respectful intention.

Assessing a Yes, Maybe, or No Answer

Now that you've done the asking in this process, how can you know what your dog's response is? The shortest answer to this question is: Pay attention. Dogs are good communicators, especially if they do *not* want Reiki. You'll know what they want if you are paying attention. But be careful. It's best not to get too set on what dogs are *supposed* to do during treatments; every treatment is different because every dog will choose to receive Reiki in his or her own way.

You must abide by what your dog decides, even if it is not the answer you were hoping for. If your dog says "no" to a treatment, you must respect that. If your dog says "yes" to a treatment, you can then proceed to connect, offering them whatever energy they are open to receiving. If your dog says, "Maybe. I'm not sure," that's okay, too. You can simply sit quietly in the energetic space that will be created through your intention and focus, allowing your dog to experience the energy and take a little bit if he or she wants to.

Keeping this in mind, the following are three usual signs that your animal has said "yes" or "maybe" to the treatment (which means it's okay for you to proceed):

- The dog's behavior shows interest in or appreciation of your presence. This interest will usually evolve into relaxation (such as yawning, deep relaxed breathing, sleeping, and so on).
- The dog's behavior shows an ebb and flow movement coinciding with periods of rest, relaxation, and interest in or appreciation of your presence. The dog may come to and from your hands, walking away, then coming back, lying down to rest, then getting up, and so on. This pattern may repeat many times within the course of one 30-minute session.

- As you notice that the dog seems appreciative of your presence, you will begin to feel relaxation within yourself, as well as heat, pulsing, or buzzing in your hands, arms, body, or head. This indicates an energetic connection with your dog. The periods of deeper connection will often echo the periods of deeper relaxation you observe in the dog; conversely, when the energy feels less strong within yourself, you may notice more movement and alertness in the dog.

As mentioned, in rare cases, a dog may choose to reject a Reiki treatment. He or she will display behavior such as annoyance, aggravation, and/or nervousness at your presence, along with an inability to settle. The inability to settle is always present when a dog says "no" to Reiki. Some dogs will appear nervous or annoyed about your presence at first simply because they have abuse/trauma issues in their past, but they will relax into the treatment once they realize you will not force anything on them and remain respectful of their wishes.

Sometimes when a dog says "no" to Reiki, it's not "no" forever; it's just "not right now." Your dog may just not be in the mood at that moment, and if you respect his wishes and walk away, he will probably be open to the possibility another time. Trust your gut feelings here. If you are concerned that a dog is not comfortable with Reiki, it's best to leave and try another time.

Accepting Your Dog's Answer

No matter how much you love your dog, you cannot do the healing for him. Each being on this planet, whether human or animal, is responsible for his or her own healing process. Each of us is on our own journey and has our own healing challenges throughout this life. Each of us also has our own way and time for self-healing.

You've probably met people who do everything "big." Big emotions, big highs, big lows, and when they have health issues, they have dramatic healing responses—big healing reactions! And then you know people who are more reserved and inward in everything they do: measured and cautious in emotions, interactions, and also in healing. Everything is gradual, quiet, and gently done.

Well, dogs are like people in this respect. Some will say, "Bring on the energy!" and can have a quick amazing response to just one treatment. Another dog might say, "I'm not sure, let me try a little healing today," then show a very slow and gradual healing response over a longer period of time. One healing style is not better than another; it simply reflects the authentic nature of the dog in his own process—a beautiful thing to observe and support.

Once you let go of the idea that you are the "healer" of the dog, it takes the pressure off. You don't even have to worry about what the problem is; you can just offer the energy. On the other hand, you can't take any credit for the healing when it takes place, either. Instead, you might say to the dog, "Good for you. I'm so glad to see you healing yourself right now."

Being Rather Than Doing

To reiterate the most important component of this whole healing process: You, as the facilitator of the energy, do *not* actually *do* the healing—the dog does his or her own self-healing. You can only offer support, extend a healing embrace, and build a bridge of energetic balance. The dog then decides whether he or she wishes to receive energy, and how much.

After spending some time asking permission (beginner Reiki), offering Reiki (intermediate Reiki), and assessing your dog's response, you will become much more comfortable in sensing the energy and connecting with your dog. You will also become an advanced student in the language of energy. It becomes easier to accept whatever answer your dog is giving you without pushing your own agenda. At this stage, you can begin to play with the idea of letting go of offering energy and instead just sit with your dog in the energy, in the moment. In essence, you open to just "being" Reiki *with* your dog, rather than "doing" Reiki *to* your dog.

At this stage, it no longer matters who is the giver and who is the receiver: You have reached a deeper level of connection. You begin to feel a oneness with your dog, as if there were no separation. In this beautiful space even intention will fall away: You will simply open to the energy and be filled by it. You will at once go inward to your true nature and expand outward to connect with your dog. It is very difficult to describe but wonderful to experience. You and your dog will be healed and more deeply bonded as a result of this connection.

CASE HISTORY

Canine Teacher: Kirra

Reiki Practitioner: Kimberly Swan

Challenge: Nine-year-old greyhound rescue dog won't accept Reiki.

When Reiki practitioner Kimberly Swan first learned Reiki, she was, in her own words, "very zealous in doing Reiki to everyone, whether they wanted it or not." Every time Kimberly would decide to do Reiki with her dog, Kirra, the dog would give her a look that could "kill." She wanted nothing to do with the treatments. For a long time, Kimberly completely gave up even offering Reiki to Kirra. After more than a year had passed, Kimberly tried a new approach: She asked permission and left it up to Kirra whether she wanted to receive the treatment or not. Kirra immediately accepted. Through asking permission first, Kimberly was able to offer regular Reiki sessions to Kirra. She says, "Now the look on her face during her Reiki is always a sleepy smile."

Canine Lesson: Always ask permission.

CHAPTER 9

Golden Rule No. 2: Embrace Your Dog's Movement

Calm in quietude is not real calm.
When you can be calm in the midst of activity,
this is the true state of nature.

　　—Huanchu Daoren

When I first began offering Reiki to animals, naturally I followed my human ideas of what a treatment *should* look like. I would sit next to my dog and move through a series of hand positions, one after the other, starting at the head and moving toward the tail. Or I would just put my hands on the area I knew needed healing and would "send" Reiki to that area.

Very soon I realized that many dogs were displeased with certain positions, while others didn't like being touched at all. Some would settle very nicely, then when I moved my hands would become disturbed and give me an annoyed look. Sometimes, the dog's person would tell me to work on a certain area, but the dog would present another area to me instead.

This would throw me at first, and I would resist, holding onto the idea of what the dog's person had told me. Sometimes, I would physically turn the dog back around or move to the other side of the animal in order to proceed with my own ideas of how the treatment should go. Typically, the dog would disconnect at this point and walk away, ending the treatment.

Sometimes, I would put a dog on a leash so that I could make sure I covered all hand positions on the body without being disturbed by his movements. Dogs who were restrained sometimes settled into the treatment, but many times just pulled and squirmed, causing me to end the treatment. Small dogs that I put into my lap might jump down after just a few minutes and run from the room. I'd read somewhere that this means they just "don't need more than a minute or two" of Reiki. This didn't make sense to me since I still saw big issues with these dogs that needed healing. I sensed that it wasn't that they were already healed, or that they simply didn't want healing; it seemed that they just weren't open to the process—at least in the way I had presented it to them.

Knowing that more Reiki was what these dogs needed, but wondering how I could gain their acceptance, I began to question my approach. At that point, I had two choices: stick with my current ideas about what a Reiki treatment was "supposed" to entail (from a human perspective) and, therefore, basically give up, or ask them what would be acceptable to them in order to be able to create a Reiki connection and level of trust that would really last and thus support the duration of their healing process.

As I detailed in the previous chapter, once I realized that permission was needed from the animal before I could begin, the next step was realizing that restraining the animal was not working. I began to allow animals freedom of movement dur-

TRY THIS
Movement Awareness

Choose a relaxing space where you can spend an hour connecting with your dog without speaking and just being together. Go outdoors, if possible, such as into your yard, where you will be closer to nature's energy. Allow yourself to let go of thoughts and daily con-cerns, and focus on just connecting with your dog. You may want to pet your dog or just sit near him.

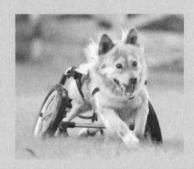

Allow your dog to determine what, if any, physical movement happens within the space. If he moves away, try following him and see what happens. Also try mirroring his movements to see the responses. For example, move away if he moves away; move closer when he moves closer. Try sitting still in the center of the space, ignoring his movements and see your dog's response. Some dogs are very high energy and active, while others are more sedentary. Some are very sensitive to our every movement, while others don't take much notice.

This is a great exercise in being with a dog on his own terms. When you do this, you can begin to feel each dog's unique sensitivities and preferences. You'll also begin to see how your own physical movement and presence affects your dog's movements and ability to relax. Your dog's natural energy level will mostly determine how much movement you will see during Reiki, but you can sometimes assist a dog in relaxing by choosing respectful and nondominant, noninvasive body language.

ing treatment, so when I treated dogs, I would simply sit with them in the middle of a room where they could move around.

Over time, I began to see a typical pattern of movement back and forth from my hands; I found that if I just picked a spot in the general vicinity where the animal was and allowed the energy to flow, the animal would usually spend some time near my hands and some time at a distance from me. Sometimes I got the best response when I would mirror their movements with my own. An animal would move away and I would also; when they moved toward me, I, too, would move toward them. This happened with dogs, cats, horses, small animals, and even wild animals over and over again.

Soon I began to discover that an interesting piece of the healing puzzle began to fall into place. When I didn't "do" certain hand positions, but instead allowed the animals to come to me or just observed their behavior and offered healing from a distance, the animals would more often than not actually show me the areas that needed healing. Sometimes these were the areas I expected and sometimes not. Some animals would put a sore or hurting paw or joint into my hands. Emotionally distraught animals would place their heads or chests into my hands. Other animals would show me from a distance by holding up a limb toward me, stomping a foot, or turning around and positioning an area of the body toward me. I found that the less I interfered with the animal's movement during the treatment, the more aware I became of their issues and the healing effects Reiki was having. This was quite a turnaround, as I had initially gotten my best intuitive feedback through feeling the energy with the animals directly under my hands.

TRY THIS
Healing Pond
(special thanks to Joyce Leonard for this beautiful imagery)

Set aside 20 to 30 minutes. As you set your intention to offer healing to your dog, imagine you can pour all your light and love—your compassionate intention—into a pond. Imagine your dog can drink from this healing pond as they wish and as they are comfortable. This is a great way to practice nondominant thinking, where we leave the whole process up to our dog (rather than taking over with "you need this!" thinking). The more gentle and open we can be with our thoughts as we connect to our dogs for healing, the better responses we will receive from them.

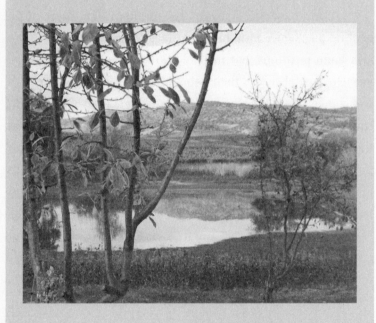

At the same time, I began to realize that animals seemed able to respond well to the treatment even if they moved the whole time. In other words, animals didn't need to lie motionless for an hour in order to show healing improvements. In fact, with some animals that I had formerly restrained during treatment, I saw a much deeper level of relaxation and acceptance of the Reiki when they were able to move freely. Freedom of movement, for me, became the natural second step after to asking permission/offering Reiki/being Reiki. How can we really be leaving it up to the animal's choice if we have certain specific expectations about how they should behave during the treatment?

In a nutshell, when we learn to embrace our dog's movement, when we allow the treatment to unfold each time as it does naturally, without worry, what we are really doing is letting go of our wishes, hopes, and beliefs about what the treatment should look like or how they should react to the energy.

Yes, human Reiki treatments are still and quiet (for the most part). Yes, *we* like to lie down on a massage table for an hour when we receive Reiki. But we are humans, not dogs. In other words, embracing movement during Reiki is a way to learn to meet our dogs in the energy on their own canine terms, without judgment and preconception, and with respect for who they are and how they process healing.

CASE HISTORY

Canine Teacher: Lady

Reiki Practitioner: Joe Polivick

Challenge: Rescued German shepherd must overcome "crippling shyness" with people in order to be able to find a forever home.

Joe remembers his first introduction to Lady, a German shepherd who had been rescued from a backyard breeder's property, where she had lived her life on a chain. When he entered her kennel, she "sank down on all fours and hid her head between her paws."

Joe began by offering Reiki to Lady outside her kennel. After a few sessions, he began to offer Reiki inside a small private room at the shelter, so that Lady could move freely. Each session she relaxed more, learning to trust Joe little by little. During her last Reiki session (before she was placed in her new foster home), Lady was lying closely to Joe, completely relaxed. Her foster home reported that Lady was a "gem" and adapted easily to living in her new home. In Joe's words, "Reiki was the key that opened the door to Lady's heart."

Lesson: Allowing dogs to move freely during sessions builds trust quickly between practitioner and dog so that healing can take place.

CHAPTER 10

Golden Rule No. 3: Let Go of Your Hands

Don't seek, don't search, don't ask, don't knock, don't demand—relax.
If you relax, it comes. If you relax, it is there.
If you relax, you start vibrating with it.

　—Osho

I once visited a Japanese garden that had a beautiful koi pond. It was very large, and I sat down several feet from the edge and quietly observed the fish. They were keeping to themselves in the shade, along the opposite bank. I quietly sat in the lotus position, closed my eyes, and began offering Reiki. I felt a strong flow of energy that felt like pulsing throughout my hands and arms. Without even opening my eyes, I knew someone in that pond was happy to accept the treatment!

A few moments later, a large splash startled me (and soaked me through!). One of the biggest koi had swum over to the edge nearest where I was sitting, jumped high out of the water, and splashed me with a big slap of his tail on the surface. I had opened my eyes just in time to see him retreating beneath the surface of the water again. What an amazing experience that was! This was a good reminder that you don't need to have direct physical contact to connect strongly with another being energetically.

In a human Reiki treatment, the client will lie down, fully clothed, on a massage table (or sometimes sit in a chair) for an hour or so while the practitioner goes through a series of light hand positions on certain parts of the body. Because we associate our hands with a variety of "pushing" and "pulling" activities throughout our lives, it is natural to assume that with Reiki, our hands are "doing" some healing to the person, or directing the flow of energy within the client in some way—certain hand positions may appear to correspond to "sending" energy to a certain physical area. This is not always the case, however.

This is because Reiki practitioners do not control energy flow within the pathways and meridians of the client. They do not "unblock" a certain area or "heal" a particular issue. Practitioners may be aware of a certain area that needs healing and place their hands over or near the area, but what the energy decides to do and where it is actually going are not within the practitioner's control.

Hands are, for humans, a primary way to connect with the world. We depend on our hands for so many things. When we begin learning this new and subtle language of energy, it is natural for us to depend upon our hands and the sensitivities in them to help us to sense the energy. It's good to remember, and dogs are a great example of this, that hands are only a very surface way to communicate with the world. If we want to be successful in working with dogs and energy, we just need to learn to go deeper.

It is also natural for us to have preconceptions about healing and physical contact. It is just part of our own life experience. Petting, hugging, and snuggling our dogs certainly provide wonderful feelings of stress relief and relaxation for both us and them. And when we think of healing treatments of any kind—be they visits to a conventional doctor or acupuncture or chiropractic appointments—certain preconceptions from our past experiences come to mind. Whether they were human treatments or those given to our dogs, we probably remember an exam or massage table inside a small examination room and a certain amount of time where we (or our dog) sat or lay down to receive the treatment from the doctor or practitioner.

This is the interesting thing about Reiki—and one of its challenges: What appears to be happening on the surface and what is actually happening on the deeper healing levels are often two very different things. In our hope to help the dog who may be sick, it is easy to let our ego take over and try to assert some control over what is happening—to, in other words, "fix" the problem with our "healing hands."

As I have mentioned, in the early days of my practice, there were many times dogs would walk away when I would approach them for Reiki (this walk would sometimes turn into a run if I followed them), but I began to notice that they would often come back to me if I stayed where I was and didn't follow their retreat. I wondered what would happen if I avoided this chase/retreat ritual altogether and, instead of approaching them, just sat nearby and began the treatment.

I noticed that when I didn't approach them physically at all, dogs would react favorably to my presence and would respond quickly and openly to the energy I offered. When I would start treatments from 5 to 10 feet away (or more) and just allow them to continue to move around, not worrying about what they were doing, they would usually relax very quickly. Some dogs would actually come to me and put certain body parts (often the parts I knew were hurting, like a sore joint or paw) right into my hands. But other dogs actually avoided my hands, especially on their injured areas.

For example, a dog who had hip dysplasia might offer me his head. Regardless of my physical interaction with the dogs, I saw wonderful healing results when they were able to relax into the treatment. In other words, it appeared that the relaxation of the dog (showing the openness of the dog to the Reiki) rather than the physical contact given seemed to indicate whether a treatment was successful or not.

As a beginner in this process, I didn't at first feel the energy as easily when I sat at some distance from the dog, so I wondered if the treatments I gave from a distance were somehow inferior to the treatments where the dogs allowed me physical contact. The more treatments I carried out, however, the more I began to see that it didn't matter whether my hands made physical contact with the area that was hurting the dog; if I made a good connection, with the dog his health issues improved. In fact, I began to witness some of the best results in treatments where the dogs never came over to me at all! As a result of these many healing experiences, along with the dogs' increasing acceptance of my presence when I did not approach them, I began to let go of my need to put my hands on them. I became comfortable with the movement they showed during treatments. As a natural consequence of this lessening of reliance on my hands, I suppose, I began to envision Reiki creating more of a general healing space outward from my entire body, rather than a specific beam of energy out of my hands.

I watched time and again as animals relaxed into this space of Reiki and healed themselves. With practice, I began to be able to sense the energetic connection between the dog and me, even when we were at some distance from each other. Over time and with more experience, the proximity, direction, and position of my hands became, for me, nonissues.

We humans like the feel of physical contact—we've all heard of the power of healing touch—so it makes a lot of sense that touch can have an important place in the human Reiki treatment, from both the perspectives of the practitioner and client. Working with dogs is different. Some prefer hands-on contact, but many do not. Honoring this difference and respecting dogs for their sensitivities is key to being successful in offering Reiki.

After completing a Reiki assignment for one of my classes, where he was required to offer Reiki to his dog from across the room (rather than with the dog in his lap), a student once complained to me, "I see your point about not touching the animal and all, but actually, it's easier for me to sense the energy when my hands are on her."

My response was, "Yes, we are human. I am sure that it *is* easier for you. But remember, it's not about you; it's about your dog."

This was quite an eye-opener for the student, and he began having more success once he began practicing letting go of his hands. The interesting part was that he had originally contacted me because of his frustration that his animal didn't seem open to Reiki. How easy it is for humans to get lost in our own perspective. We get so wrapped up in our own understanding and experience of what is happening or not happening that we almost forget the animal! But luckily, it's also easy for our dogs to help us find our way again—if we are open to hearing what they are telling us, that is.

Reiki practitioners use compassionate intention to support the dog. The dog, however, has complete control of the session, deciding how much energy to receive and where the energy goes. This is often not a conscious process for the dog as receiver of the energy. So how does this happen above and beyond the mind's understanding and awareness?

Reiki helps to induce and support relaxation and stress relief, which are the optimal conditions for self-healing. So in a way, you could say that Reiki helps to "switch on" the body's ability to self-heal.

Because of the ritualized movement of hand positions in human Reiki treatments, it's easy to fool ourselves into believing that we are somehow controlling the healing process, "sending" energy with our hand positions "here" and "there." In reality, hand positions have nothing whatsoever to do with the deeper process of healing. Hands are a very superficial way for humans to connect to energy when we are first learning. The true power of energy, however, lies in the ability to completely let go of our reliance on our hands and allow the

TRY THIS
Healing Heart, Healing Breath

Sit at some distance from your dog. Feel your roots going deep into the earth and earth energy coming up your roots into your heart center. Place your hands in *gassho* (palms together, in front of your heart). On the in breath, bring white healing light up from the earth through the base of your spine and on up to your heart. On the out breath, expand the energy out of your heart, creating a space of light and healing all around you. Continue this in-and-out breathing pattern for several minutes. You can keep your hands in *gassho* or slowly open your palms and face them outward in an expansive way. Imagine that your dog can "step in" and "step out" of the healing heart space you have created at his own discretion. Use your breath simply to hold the space and offer the possibility. After a few minutes, return your breathing to normal, rest your hands on your lap, and sit in the energy you have created for another 20 to 30 minutes. Watch your dog for signs of relaxation and connection with you.

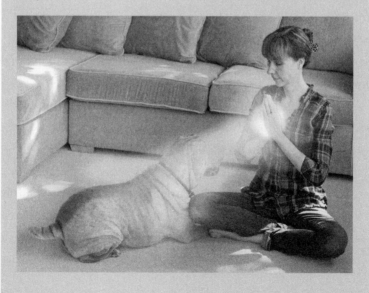

energy to flow throughout our entire body. More than that, we must learn to allow the energy to flow even deeper—beyond our physical bodies and into our minds and spirits.

We might think of our energetic existence as consisting of the following:

- A fragile, mortal, physical layer on the outside—the layer that is easiest to see and understand;
- A complex mental/emotional layer beneath the physical, which takes more work to recognize and communicate with;
- And finally, a spiritual layer in the deepest core of our being that goes on infinitely. For some, this is very difficult to sense and know during our lifetime, yet we all merge completely into this layer when we die.

The deepest healing we can experience occurs on all three levels at once because we are composed of more than just a body, more than just a mind, more than just a spirit. The harmony and balance of all these parts is what allows individual healing.

Letting go of our reliance on physical touch helps us remember the profound totality of our essence as spiritual beings. It is very important to understand when offering Reiki to dogs, because they share the same essence as us. The more we let go of the physical, the easier it will be to sense and be in touch with deeper energetic connections and healing. When we open to this level of communication—being and healing—it becomes much easier to support our dogs.

CASE HISTORY

Canine Teacher: Teddy

Reiki Practitioner: Janice Mitchell

Challenge: Rescued Shetland sheepdog is terrified of people.

When Janice first met Teddy, he had just been rescued from the home of a hoarder and was huddled in the back of his kennel, "scared and filthy." Janice sat in meditation pose outside his kennel and, as she began offering Reiki, whispered to Teddy that he had the choice to "accept the healing energy or not."

After several minutes, Janice noticed something amazing: The rest of the kennels had gone silent—completely and totally silent! Teddy was now away from the corner of the kennel, watching her intently. Janice decided to finish her treatment from inside the kennel. After just a few moments, Teddy came forward, first lying down right in front of Janice, then giving a huge sigh of relief and relaxation.

After this, Janice was able to place Teddy quickly in a foster home that could work on his socialization skills. When she went to visit him, she sat down nearby and began offering Reiki. Almost immediately, she remembers, Teddy "locked his little brown eyes on me as if to say, 'I know that energy!' He then slowly came within two feet of me and stood there for his Reiki." The healing process had truly begun!

Lesson: Since it works well from a distance, Reiki is ideal for use with dogs who have issues with physical touch.

CASE HISTORY

Canine Teacher: Ottway

Reiki Practitioner: Annamaria Mayes

Challenge: A two-year-old rescued lurcher is malnourished and anxious.

When Annamaria first met Ottway, he was in his shelter kennel, continually jumping and running in circles, "too nervous to sit or eat." To build trust with Ottway, Annamaria took him to a small private room within the shelter and decided to show him what Reiki looked like by giving herself a Reiki treatment while he watched. Although her eyes were closed, Annamaria could hear Ottway regularly pausing in front of her during his nervous walk. As she finished her treatment he finally sat down on the blanket in front of her. She gently put her hands on his shoulders and chest as he finally relaxed into a hands-on Reiki treatment.

Annamaria remembers that special treatment, saying, "Ottway closed his eyes and quickly entered a deep Reiki sleep, often sighing profusely, sometimes twitching and, most importantly, completely undisturbed by outside noises." As she took him back to his kennel, she could already see the improvement and relaxation in his behavior. A few weeks later, Ottway found his forever home.

Lesson: Once again, always allow the dog to choose, and it's best to start treatments hands-off until the dog initiates hands-on.

CHAPTER 11

Golden Rule No. 4: Release Expectations

Some of us think holding on makes us strong;
but sometimes it is letting go.

  −Herman Hesse

Reiki with our dogs is really about connecting from a space of compassion. It's about wanting to help, but at the same time being open to the process (and the unknown) and trusting whatever happens—letting go of expectations and releasing our human desire to control the situation and the outcome of the treatment.

This is not always easy, especially when we are working with a dog with whom we have especially close emotional ties. It's a lesson in what true compassion for another being is all about. It's about surrender—surrender to the universal flow, the ebb and flow of existence that creates balance through change. When we can surrender to this reality, we can go deeper into the essence of compassion, and in so doing become more effective at facilitating and supporting the balanced space that helps us truly heal.

As I've mentioned previously, healing is sometimes a bit of a mystery. Sometimes, I'll go to a treatment thinking the animal needs one thing, and something altogether different is healed. Other times, I'll go in thinking that I am the "practitioner," then the animal offers me a powerful gift and I find myself wondering, Hey, who's healing whom?

In my experience, the best way to facilitate this beautiful and profound healing energy is simply to be part of the flow. As my teacher Frans Stiene says, the ideal state during a Reiki treatment is for your mind to be a blank sheet of paper. As facilitators of this process, we do not do anything except allow the energy to flow through us. In finding the courage to let go, we come back to our souls and touch the ultimate truth of why we are here in the first place—to help each other.

For some dogs, healing means a physical recovery. For others, healing means a rejuvenation in spirits and emotions before the dog passes away. Over the years I've worked with Reiki, I've learned that the process of healing is not so simple to explain. But I trust that healing does happen on one level or another—just not always the way I'd envisioned.

The healing that Reiki facilitates is often deeper than just changes that can be seen, so it helps to let go of our expectations if we are to open to these more subtle shifts in a dog's being. We may be doing Reiki for a dog's physical problem, yet begin to see emotional healing or amazing changes in the attitude of that dog. For example, it's common to see the unlikeliest of animals become open to connecting with humans during and immediately after treatment. An abused dog that has completely shut down to the world may begin to wag his tail with delight at the first feeling of Reiki energy. A depressed and withdrawn dog who usually curls up motionless in the corner may begin to come forward for petting just after a treatment.

Often I'm asked to work with animals that have physical issues (as humans we tend to see and concern ourselves with the problems and symptoms easily seen with our eyes). But more often than not, there is an emotional origin that Reiki can touch, and once this process begins to unfold, it often seems there is no stopping it!

Being able to make positive connections with animals who have given up all trust in humans due to past abuse and trauma is an incredible feeling. It's amazing to see the dog's heart open and his emotions start to heal. Once this happens, the physical symptoms heal soon after, and the animal's entire being begins to move toward balance.

Many people seek out Reiki because their dog is dying and they hope that Reiki will heal the dog's body. Sometimes this happens and more time is given; often, though, we discover many other gifts of healing along the road to the end-of-life transition instead.

On a physical level, it is common for dogs to receive a certain level of healing of their physical symptoms, so that the time they have left is much more comfortable. For example, the dog's appetite often returns, his breathing becomes easier, his mobility improves, his digestion rebalances, his blood work improves, and so on. In other words, although the underlying disease may still be present, the dog can, with the support of Reiki, experience a profound relief of symptoms.

Supporting our dogs in their transitional process forces us to face our fears and beliefs about our own mortality. The more we can connect with our animals energetically as they approach their deaths, the more we can connect with healing possibilities not only for them but also for ourselves. We unexpectedly find ourselves assisting not only our animals but also ourselves, and this self-support in turn helps our dogs in their own journeys. In addition, confronting and learning to release our own fears about dying allows us to be truly present for those who are transitioning.

We must work toward an evolution in our consciousness. This requires becoming aware that our compassionate intention, together with our openness and surrender to the energy around us, can bring about change just as surely as our physical actions can. Once we realize this, it can be extremely empowering. No longer do we have to sit by helplessly when an animal we love is ill, injured, or in need. We can assist them.

But along with this new knowledge of the power of our compassion—the power of energy—comes a humbling realization: We actually have no control over the outcomes of situations, and we cannot direct this limitless universal energy; we can only facilitate its higher work.

It seems the energy of the universe operates according to certain laws of existence, although we have yet to know and understand what those laws are. (I'm counting on *you*, all you quantum physicists out there, to discover the answers!) In observing life and time evolving through nature's cycles, we can see that all things move out of and back into balance through change. We can find inner harmony and peace through our surrender to, acceptance of, and comfort with the inevitability of this change. Through our work with animals, we see that although we may observe a particular need in an animal, we may also observe the animal sensing the goodness, comfort, and power of the energy we are offering them—coming to us as if attracted to a magnet by the energy itself.

Still, the unfolding healing process is itself mysterious and operates beyond our conscious understanding. Rather than desperately push for our desires, we must learn to sit back and allow the universe to flow through us. In so doing, we become agents for balance through change—for the harmony and peace that are the inevitable results of true healing.

I've found that clinging to my small and personal understanding of the dog, the healing issue, the situation, and my own desire for an outcome actually inhibits my ability to "get in that space" where Reiki (and thus healing) can flow purely and strongly. I can get in my own way, so to speak. Thoughts are very powerful, so when we are thinking *so* strongly about

TRY THIS
Holding an Intention of No Expectations

When offering energy, remain neutral in your observation of how the treatment unfolds. Hold the intention that the energy flows freely to the room and anyone who wants it, and that it doesn't matter to you who takes it, how they take it, how long it lasts, and so on. In other words, try to be completely neutral about your expectations for when and how the treatment unfolds. Hold this focus briefly before beginning a treatment and revisit it whenever you find yourself placing your own wishes and hopes onto how an animal should behave during a treatment.

what we want to happen with a dog, we are focused on pushing energy in one direction, rather than allowing it to flow unimpeded to balance and harmony. The reality is that whether we push and pull, this way and that, with our thoughts (I want *this* to happen; I wish for *that* to occur), the dog's journey is his own, and we cannot control another's destiny.

TRY THIS
Vessel of Light

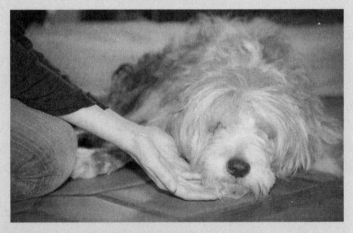

As you offer your animal healing energy, mentally step back from your own understanding of the things that need healing. See yourself as an empty vessel, ready to be filled with the universal light and wisdom of the healing energy of the universe. See this energy filling your entire being and aura with white light, flowing and working for your dog's highest good, which is beyond your own conscious understanding. Empty your mind of worries, concerns, and control issues. Open yourself to becoming one with the energy of highest good moving first through you, then to the animal's areas of need. Hold this emptiness and relaxed state of mind as the energy flows for several minutes at a time.

It's about realizing the illusion. To be successful practitioners of Reiki, we have to wrap our minds around two important facts: the awesome power of the energy we are working with and our passive role in the healing process. Once we do that, we can truly connect and see the wonders of Reiki play out before our eyes.

When we release our expectations, we also find it easier to be open to the possibility that our dogs may be helping us just as much as we are helping them. The more we connect with them, the more we realize that this whole healing space into which we are diving is a two-way exchange. We are offering healing, yet we'll often feel ourselves being healed. We are supporting change in our dogs, yet we are often changed. We are creating a space of balance for the dog, yet are supported in our own journeys toward balance.

With the benefit of time and experience, it becomes apparent that the animals themselves play an active role in all of this. As we learn to speak the language of energy, we'll become aware that although the energetic nuances may be subtle to us, they are clear and obvious to our dogs. At first, we may struggle to feel what is going on, but the dogs feel it easily and show us what's going on through their behavior. We may wonder, Is anything happening? Then we observe our dog's response and realize, yes, without a doubt, something is shifting.

When we release expectations, it becomes easier to notice that we can help more dogs and other animals around us than just the ones on which we initially focus. When we open ourselves up to the animals, direct our hearts and minds toward their welfare, and commit ourselves to daily Reiki practice, they will be drawn to our energy. We may begin to notice that every day, expectedly and unexpectedly, animals literally "appear." Domesticated and wild, affectionate and fearful, enthusiastic and cautious: The animals will find us.

At first we may think that they have come to us for healing, since we have set our compassionate intention to support them, and, in fact, that may be a piece of the story. But we may also begin to see certain patterns in the kinds of issues we support them in with Reiki that reveal something in ourselves that needs healing—issues that are mirrored in ourselves, that we, too, need to work on.

And as the animals heal through the Reiki connection, so too will we heal. A horse's deep sigh and muzzle resting upon my chest as I struggle with grief; a dog's gentle paw upon my hand when I feel alone; a cat curling up to purr atop my aching stomach—yes, the animals are aware of our healing issues and are happy to support us. In surrendering ourselves to the process—whatever it looks like for our dogs—we are opening ourselves to a deeper awareness of compassion, not only with them but also with nature and all of existence. When we are in this space, there are no boundaries, no limitations, no time, no space—no "me" and no "you."

To support our healing journey, it is helpful to study and practice all the elements of the system of Reiki by finding a human Reiki teacher to support our practice, as well as sit with the animals and share their energy. Of course, this daily Reiki "practice," this study of a system of techniques, is not required for our dogs; they do not need to work at connecting—for most of them, it's just who they are and where they live every day. This is why they are so easily able to be "Man's Best Friend," supporting us in our lives, assisting us in our work, and helping us to heal. It's also why they are so appreciative when we come to them openly and simply from a space of compassion and surrender.

CASE HISTORY

Canine Teacher: Lucky

Reiki Practitioner: Shelly Hughes

Challenge: Six-year-old black Labrador is diagnosed with a large tumor, encompassing his esophagus, lungs, and kidneys.

When Shelly first met Lucky after his diagnosis, she was told that he hadn't eaten in three days. After an hour-long session of Reiki, he started eating! The next day, he also was able to eat. For his next treatment, Lucky came forward and offered his neck and chest to Shelly. She placed her hands there, and he wagged his tail to let her know that was just right. Once when she tried to move her hands, he put his paw over Shelly's hands to let her know not to move.

By the end of the treatment he had fallen into a deep sleep. Shelly said she felt a strong connection with him that was "quite wonderful." A few days later, Lucky made his transition, but in Shelly's words, "What a privilege and great honor it was to have known and offered Reiki to Lucky. I was glad I was able to give him some comfort in his final days. He was surely a true friend and loyal companion."

Lesson: Reiki has the beautiful ability to offer peace and relaxation to a dog in his final days.

CASE HISTORY

Canine Teacher: Winnie

Reiki Practitioner: Kathy Tracy

Challenge: Golden retriever is diagnosed with cancer.

Winnie joined Kathy's family as a four-month-old puppy and spent 11 years as part of her family. In Winnie's later years, although she slowed down, she never gave any indication that anything serious was going on. When Kathy learned Reiki, Winnie became her teacher. Kathy says, "When I doubted myself and wondered if I was 'doing it right,' her patient and peaceful spirit told me that all was well." Each evening, Kathy would offer her Reiki, and she just "soaked it up!" As Kathy remembers, "She enjoyed hands-on treatments—but 'goldens' always enjoy hands-on anything!"

One day Winnie wasn't feeling well, so off to the vet she went. The vet recommended exploratory surgery to try to determine what the problem was. "Before the surgery, she was like her old self!" says Kathy. "She even tried to jump up on our daughter and give her a hug when she saw her. We were with her as she was anesthetized, and I was convinced that everything was going to be fine and that we would be taking her home. Then the doctor called me into surgery when Winnie was on the table. Her liver was completely black. Then the doctor explained that the rest of the organs were also eaten up with cancer. In addition, there was a huge mass in her intestines."

Kathy and her family made the difficult decision to euthanize Winnie. Kathy shares, "I'm convinced that Reiki was responsible for making Winnie's life pain-free during her last few months, and my family and I will be eternally grateful for that. Her teachings live on with me, and I hope I can share that gift with other animals."

Lesson: No matter how severe the illness, Reiki can help sustain a good quality of life in the final days.

CHAPTER 12

Golden Rule No. 5: Always See the Positive

A bug on a branch
Swept away down the river
Still singing his song.

  —Issa

The positive thinker sees the invisible, feels the
intangible, and achieves the impossible.

  —Anonymous

As we have discussed earlier, Reiki goes where it needs to go to support balance and create healing possibilities in the dogs with whom we work. We can never give too much Reiki because dogs will only take what they need. So then we can't really do it wrong, can we?

Well, not exactly. You can't give "bad" Reiki or cause harm to an animal through the Reiki process, but, as I've illustrated in the several previous chapters, our approach as a human being is very important. We are offering the possibility of healing to our dogs, but we need to remember they aren't just accepting Reiki; they're accepting a connection with us, as facilitators of the Reiki process. Because dogs are so attuned to our states of being, it is really important that we are in the "right space," so to speak, within our own attitudes and bodies. Most importantly, we should be in a positive frame of mind during treatment. When we approach them with positivity, we will receive a much deeper trust and openness to the healing of Reiki than we ever could otherwise.

Sometimes, the dogs we work with are facing tremendous healing challenges and crises. They may be shelter animals who endured years of neglect and abuse, or loved family animals who are facing death, with grieving family members all around them. When we arrive on the scene to offer Reiki, we have a very important role to play. We are there to be the beacon of light, love, peace, and pure positivity that the animals (and their people) can hold onto. We must be able to hold this possibility of balance and healing potential within ourselves first, if we are to help others.

It doesn't help dogs (not to mention their people) if we pity them for their pasts, feel uncomfortable with the physical ailments they show, or fear the deaths they may imminently face. Not only will these attitudes not help, they will actually hinder our ability to help them.

Being the sensitive creatures they are, dogs are completely aware of our emotional states when we are with them. We can't hide anything from them. If we are afraid, they will know it. If we feel sad and hopeless, they will know it. If we feel sorry for them, they will feel that. This is why when we assist dogs in their healing, we will also confront our own issues.

I clearly remember the dog who taught me my most important lesson in staying positive. This dog was a pit bull whose immune system was compromised, with the result that she had broken out in sores all over her body and lost most of her fur. It was almost impossible to see what her original color must have been. Her feet were swollen to three times their normal size and were bleeding. She couldn't walk (when she did, she left bloody footprints) and was very uncomfortable.

To make matters worse, she was in a shelter with no family of her own. She was what everyone called "a tough case." None of the medicines that had been tried had had any effect on her condition, and after a few months, the veterinarian determined that if she didn't get better within a few weeks on her own, her body may not have the reserves to get well at all.

I was brought into the kennel aisle where the dog was located, given an up-to-date history, and asked to offer Reiki.

TRY THIS
Traditional Reiki Self-Healing Technique from Nentatsu Ho
(*The Reiki Sourcebook*, p. 263)

You may be seated or lying down to use this technique. Create an affirmation that you wish to use, using language that sees it as already a reality. For example, "I am filled with peace and calm." Place one hand on your forehead and the other hand at the base of your neck. Repeat your affirmation for as long as five minutes, repeating it aloud or silently in your mind. Remove your hand from your forehead while keeping the other hand on your neck for up to five minutes.

As we stood there talking about the dog, I observed some members of the public walking through the kennel, looking at all the dogs. Without fail, when someone would walk by her, he or she would have some kind of negative response: an audible exhale or sigh, a head shake, some kind of comment like, "Oh, poor thing!" or even worse, they would quickly avert their eyes and walk by as if she weren't there. Although I'm sure people didn't mean any harm, I could feel the negative thoughts and feelings being heaped upon this little dog.

As we approached her kennel, I felt intuition taking over and a strong intention of lightness and joy spread throughout my whole being. I looked at the little dog, then allowed myself to look deeper and see her inner being, her beautiful and courageous spirit. I smiled, introduced myself to her, and

TRY THIS
Technique for Visualizing Positive Outcomes

First try this technique on yourself. Pick a situation in your life that is difficult. Spend some time visualizing how it would look if it were already perfectly healed, resolved, and in perfect balance. Let yourself see all the physical details of this perfection: How does it look, sound, smell, taste? Then allow your body to feel the wonderful healing of the situation. How does your heart feel when this is perfectly resolved? Spend some time just basking in the picture and feelings of this beautiful scene.

Next, choose a health issue or situation that your animal is facing. Rather than going through all your worries and what is wrong, focus only on seeing everything as if it is perfect, in balance, and healed already. Then allow your emotions to follow your mind's eye. Bask in the joy and peace that follows from the image of perfect healing of your animal.

told her she was wonderful. And indeed she was—her external condition notwithstanding, her whole body literally wagged with sweetness.

The staff member went into her kennel, gathered her into a blanket (as she couldn't walk), and carried her to a private room where we could be alone and quiet for a Reiki treatment. After she was put down on the floor in the room, the most amazing personality emerged from this pit bull. She was gentle, loving, and happy, as if completely unaware of her physical ailments.

She already seemed to know why I was there, and before I could even ask her if she'd like Reiki, she had crawled into my lap and completely relaxed for a deep Reiki nap. As I offered the treatment, I focused my inner vision on her as already being in a perfectly balanced state. I saw her in my mind's eye as beautiful, smooth, and silky, running playfully on healed feet through endless green grass. She fell into a deep sleep for almost an hour. During this time she sighed and took deep breaths, and even ran in her dreams for part of the time!

After I left, I continued to hold the perfectly healed version of her in my mind and heart every day. Remarkably, soon after that first treatment, she began to show signs of improvement. Against all odds and after so much time, she was finally coming around! I continued to work with her each week for a few weeks. The shelter began to hold out hope that she would be able to heal. After a few weeks of Reiki, she found a foster home to give her the quiet space and attention she needed to build herself back to health. Eventually, she healed completely and found a forever home.

In looking back on this experience, I marveled at this little dog's strength to come back from such odds. I knew she could do it, and I think that knowing that she was not alone somehow helped her. Because I saw her differently from the way others viewed her, I think she trusted me. This trust allowed her to open to healing more quickly and in a deeper way than might have otherwise been possible.

After that experience, I find myself creating the place of perfection in my mind whenever I perform Reiki with dogs. If I'm with a dog who is old, infirm, and dying, I visualize his vibrant, young puppy self. If I am with an elderly dog who is struggling with arthritis, I visualize an athletic, energetic youngster. If I see a body showing injuries and scars, I visualize them as already perfectly healed. If I'm working with two animals who don't get along, I see them as perfect friends and allies. If I'm working with a dog who has an overpowering fear and anxiety of the world, I see him or her as fearless and courageous in all things.

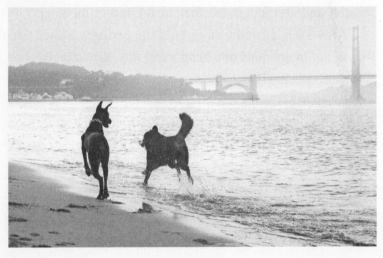

TRY THIS
Moonlight Beacon

Find a quiet space to meditate, where you will not be disturbed. Choose a comfortable place to sit, close your eyes, and take a deep breath, exhaling slowly. Imagine you are sitting on the edge of a cliff, looking out to the endless sea. It is night and very dark, except for a beautiful full moon, which illuminates the surface of the waves upon the ocean.

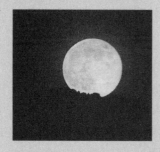

Out there somewhere in the darkness is your animal, looking for a way back to shore. Breathe earth energy up from your roots and moon energy down through your crown. Feel your body, mind, and spirit filling with the brightest moonlight of healing and harmony. Feel your entire being becoming a beacon of balance—a moon of hope and healing for your animal.

Imagine that your animal can easily follow the bright light of healing that you radiate, and if they so choose, may navigate the dark waters to perfect safety, healing, and harmony. The path to healing is easily illuminated by the moonlight; the way becomes clear. Hold this moonlight beacon within yourself for 20 to 30 minutes.

I've spent so much time in so many different situations seeing the positive with my heart that sometimes it's more difficult for me to actually see the external problems that everyone else seems to be focusing on. I encourage you to cultivate this ability to see below the surface of whatever is presented to you—to see hope, possibility, healing, and light in any situation, no matter how dark it may initially seem.

I've seen dogs respond to my positive attitude in tangible ways, with physical issues clearing and emotional distresses improving. One time, an old dog picked up a toy and brought it over to me. His person said he hadn't showed any interest in play for many months. A very fearful dog ended up in my lap by the end of the treatment—a behavior that startled and amazed his people.

Once the dogs decide I am okay, they open up with deep trust to the energy and healing possibilities Reiki offers. It's so important to communicate to animals through our minds and emotions that we believe in them, that we believe they can heal, be well, and be whole again. When they feel that we are their advocates in love and light, they will not only open to Reiki but will literally run to us for it!

I've realized over time that perfect balance is always available, and indeed always exists on some level (whether it be physical, emotional, or spiritual). It isn't for me to say what the healing for the dog will look like, but for the time I am with him, I will hold him in such love, light, peace, and harmony, nothing else matters. I create the most perfect space for them for the time that I am there. It seems that for dogs, that makes all the difference.

PART IV
The Circle of Healing

When the pupil is ready to learn, a teacher will appear.

—Zen proverb

CHAPTER 13

Opening to Receive Healing from the Animals

When I let go of what I am, I become what I might be.
—Lao Tzu

As a Reiki practitioner, I've worked with lots of different kinds of animals over the years—from well-loved family dogs, cats, and birds to sanctuary and rescue horses, elephants, and tigers with difficult pasts. Each animal has had lessons to impart. Each experience has changed me, shifted my energy. It is very humbling. I've found that one of the benefits of connecting with dogs is that it helps quiet the restless mind. Over the years, many of my students have complained that they have difficulty focusing or quieting their minds when meditating. I always say, "Try meditating with your dog."

Whether walking in nature, playing crazily outdoors, or just snuggling quietly together, our dogs help bring us into that moment, totally and completely, helping us to forget all our other worries and concerns. Through their purity of spirit and essence, they effortlessly draw us into their world, where they are totally engaged in whatever activity they are doing.

By sharing this space of enthusiastic engagement with them, we can practice going to that quiet place inside ourselves where mind clutter falls away and the energy of the now becomes accessible. It becomes easier to give up our "small mind" concerns and open to an expanded space of stillness where we can begin to go deeper beneath the surface of existence.

Offering Reiki to your dog can improve all areas of your interaction with him or her, including your relationship and communications. It reminds me of the bumper sticker that reads, "PLEASE LET ME BE THE PERSON MY DOG THINKS I AM." Our dogs can inspire us to be better people, and do better things. Learning Reiki can help us develop our ability to find the energetic place where all these wonderful possibilities exist. This is the place where we can easily deepen our bonds of healing with the dogs we love.

TRY THIS
Clarity and Wisdom Affirmation

Sit with the words "It is easy for me to find clarity and wisdom of direction in the path of action I should take for my animal's highest good" inside your heart and body for several minutes. Feel the meaning and truth of that possibility permeating your whole being. When you are ready, offer the words as a gentle, loving bridge of light from your heart to the heart of your animal. Continue holding that affirmation for several minutes, or as long as you wish.

A word about affirmations: Affirmations are very powerful tools for healing. They work best when they are repeated regularly and used often. It is also always best to visualize your affirmation as already having been achieved.

The first parts of this book focused on the ways we can help dogs—"rescue" them, so to speak, from whatever issues they are dealing with. It is humbling and gratifying to connect with animals energetically and to see the improvements they make!

The final part of this book discusses another aspect of these canine connections: the circle of healing that is created when we connect with dogs. We, too, are changed and healed within the Reiki healing process. We too receive lessons. We too peel back layers that have been covering up our true natures. We, too, learn to accept and surrender to challenges in order to overcome them. And with the quiet and steady devotion of our canines, no matter the challenges before us we find our way to healing.

I have received hundreds of e-mails from people all over the world and met countless students in my classes who credit their animals for setting them on the path of holistic healing. Many of these people did not find Reiki and the self-empowerment that goes along with it until long after their animal teacher had passed. But it was in caretaking their beloved animal that their hearts and minds opened to the miraculous nature of energy healing and their lives were forever set on a path toward change.

For many dog owners, it is not until all conventional medical therapies have run their course with their animals that they try holistic healing. As they learn more about holistic healing in general, the subject of energy healing comes up often. Well-known holistic therapies such as acupuncture and chiropractic work with blockages in an animal's energy as they relate to health and wellness. Other commonly used holistic systems, such as homeopathy and flower essences, work entirely on the energetic level. While researching different holistic therapies, many people discover Reiki for animals. Its gentle nature and powerful results, as well as its ability to work well even without physical contact, make it ideal for even the most serious cases, with the result that many people find it an attractive option. When I began building my private Reiki practice, these were the people who came to me looking for healing for their animals. They had simply run out of options. Their animal was dying or a hopeless case and, hey, Reiki couldn't hurt, right?

Right. In fact, for many of my clients, even in those early days of discovery, Reiki led to remarkable improvements in their animals' quality of life and many lived much longer than expected! And along with their animals, I began to see the dogs' people open and change, too.

By choosing to take an active role in our dogs' transitional journeys, no matter how difficult they prove to be, we open our hearts to some of life's most profound lessons and learn to be courageous. These lessons help us endure as we continue on life's journey and, indeed, help define who we are at the very deepest levels. This ability to grow and change as we walk the road of Reiki healing with our dogs is a humbling thing.

Because Reiki has its roots in Buddhism, we often hear Reiki teachers encouraging their students to "practice, practice, practice." Some of this practice involves just sitting; through sitting—on our own, and with our animals—we come

TRY THIS
Sun Illumination Meditation

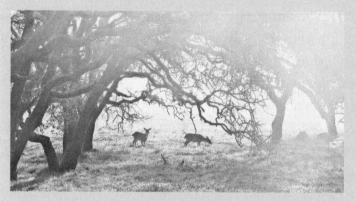

Sit in a comfortable position to meditate and close your eyes. See yourself sitting in a wide meadow in a beautiful forest. Imagine your dog is with you. The sky is cloudy and the meadow is submerged in mist, making it difficult to see. You feel that it is difficult to see what is best for your dog. Set your intention that you are open to receive whatever you need in order to know the best, wisest decision to make for your dog's highest good. Imagine that suddenly a bright ray of sunlight pierces through the mist, shining directly on you and your dog. See the clouds above you opening up and the sun's rays becoming wider and stronger. Feel the sunlight warming your body and skin. Feel its light surrounding you and expanding outward more and more.

As you breathe in, imagine the sunlight can shine even into your heart and spirit, helping you connect more deeply with your inner wisdom. See yourself and your dog, sitting in the meadow and slowly being completely (both externally and internally) engulfed in the brightest sunlight you have ever experienced. Relax for several minutes, allowing the sun to illuminate you both. Now look inside your heart. See how the sun has lit up your inner being. The answers you seek are inside you; your inner wisdom is waiting to be heard. Just take a moment to sit in the light of the sun and listen to your heart.

closer to our inner wisdom. It has been my experience that when we sit with animals, without any other purpose than just to be with them, our spiritual learning comes more quickly and easily than it does without them.

I believe this is because we are actually sitting with true spiritual masters: our energy is changed by their presence. In other words, animals assist us simply by being with us, being themselves, and sharing a connection. It is simple yet powerful. When we open ourselves up to the possibility that our dogs are not only our "fur kids" but also our spiritual teachers, our world changes and the lessons begin pouring in!

In the next few chapters, I will share stories of dogs who deepened their people's understanding of energetic wisdom, healing, and life purpose. In most cases, the beautiful gifts the animals bestowed upon these people were not actively sought; they were unexpectedly offered. Some people did not recognize the gifts they had been given until later. For all, they were life changing.

CHAPTER 14

Healing Injuries and Illness: Lessons in Courage

. . . If you are very sincere and really give up your small mind, then there is no fear and no emotional problem. Your mind is always calm, your eyes are always open, and you can hear the birds as they sing. You can see the flowers as they open. There is nothing for you to worry about. . . . We can enjoy our life fully when we understand things in this way.

—from *Not Always So* by Shunryu Suzuki

Over my years of offering Reiki treatments in animal shelters, I have seen firsthand the healing benefits for dogs in their kennels. When I arrive, the kennel is often loud, with barking, squealing, pacing, growling, and all manner of chaotic behavior going on. It is a difficult thing to sit cross-legged in the aisle of such a kennel, housing perhaps 10 to 20 dogs, and to close one's eyes and meditate; yet, this is the very practice that makes such a difference to the dogs.

After I've been meditating for several minutes, I can't count the number of times the energy in the kennels has changed: The sounds become softer, the barking reduces, and more and more dogs begin to lie or sit down to relax and look at me. In fact, on many occasions, all sound has eventually ceased and the kennels become so quiet you could hear a pin drop. It is humbling to be able to support dogs in a way that immediately and dramatically helps them—and to feel the peaceful energy that overtakes the entire kennel. Simply sitting with our dogs and meditating with them is a powerful thing.

Meditation is my solace, and I have had a daily practice for several years. I found it especially helpful while I was facing my recent treatment for breast cancer. One of the images that often came to mind in my daily meditation as I approached my surgery date was that of my dogs—Muffett, Dakota, and Mystic sitting at my feet with me as I meditated. The image was so strong and came so often that it felt for all the world that they were indeed helping me to "create a space of healing" for myself.

As I walked down the hospital corridor to the operating room and lowered myself onto the table, amid all the doctors and all that I knew was about to take place, I could feel my dearest dogs and other beloved animals (and people) with me. The peaceful blanket of Reiki embraced me, so that even at that most stressful moment, I was able to be calm.

When I returned home after a couple of days in the hospital, my puppy Mystic awaited me. Of course, she is a puppy, full of energy and bouncing around, jumping and running, as all puppies do. But her transformation as I walked slowly into

TRY THIS
Courage Affirmation

Close your eyes and sit comfortably, with the word "courage" inside your heart and body for several minutes. Feel the meaning and truth of that word/emotion permeate your whole being. Imagine what it would look like if your animal were perfectly courageous. Hold that vision, as if it is already achieved, within your heart and mind for several minutes. When you are ready, offer the possibility of courage as a gentle, loving bridge of light, from your heart to the heart of your animal. Include within the light all the emotions that go with the word. Continue holding that affirmation and bridge of light for an additional several minutes.

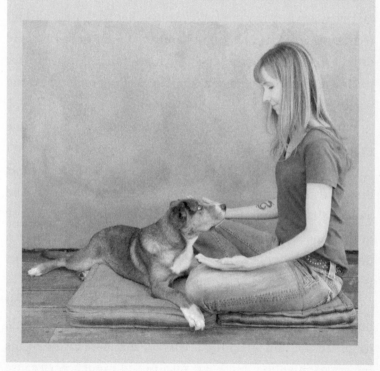

the house and gingerly sat down was something to see. Rather than greeting me roughly, she came and licked my hand and then lay down nearby with her head between her front paws, just looking up at me. She was so calm during the first weeks my recovery, in fact, that she resembled more a grown-up therapy dog than a four-month-old puppy! Her gentle presence and sweet expression as she watched me carefully those first few weeks after surgery was also, in its own way, very healing to me.

As we sat together and I healed, I remembered those few weeks after we had first adopted her, when she was very sick with giardia and coccidia. Each day she sat next to me during my meditation. She would roll over on her back with all four feet in the air. And each night before she went to bed I would offer her Reiki, and she would quickly fall fast asleep. Our path together has already been one of healing each other, and we have only been together a few months.

In reflecting on this experience, I realize that more often than not, animals find ways to heal us back, even if we don't realize it until much later. The healing they give us may be as dramatic as lowering blood pressure, healing depression, and assisting our special needs, or it could be as subtle as a nose in the hand, a kiss to the face, a quiet day on a trail, or even a dream or memory of being together. The healing of our spirits is what animals do so effortlessly.

I believe it is partly because of who they are in their bodies on this earth. Dogs are close to nature and the earth, deeper in the flow of spiritual energy, and more aware of the impact of intention and heart on life and existence. Because they live in the moment every second of every day, they have no muddiness of emotions, regrets, guilt, or masks. So when we connect in trust, love, and healing with our dog, it is like witnessing the brightest sparkling diamond of clarity, connection, and gratitude. Dogs are a shining inspiration for the way we should always be in our world.

CASE HISTORY

Canine Teacher: Sparky

Reiki Practitioner: Cathy Currea

Challenge: Nine-year-old Australian shepherd is diagnosed with lymphoma.

When Cathy came to Sparky's home to offer Reiki, the treatment lasted a little over an hour. Sparky had lumps of various sizes and shapes all over his body. The largest lump was on his left shoulder, and the two under his jaw were clearly affecting his quality of life.

After Cathy left, Sparky's person, Barbara, later reported, "We all drank a ton of water and then slept for a couple hours after you left. Funny how that happens! Sparky's lumps are all very noticeably smaller. He seems perkier but also more relaxed, if that makes sense. I think we all just plain feel better. The dogs gobbled up their dinner tonight and played together after. Thank you, thank you."

After this treatment, Sparky experienced a big improvement in symptoms for about two months. Barbara reported that the lumps in Sparky's jaw were roughly 75 percent smaller and that his energy level and appetite were greatly improved. In addition, the large lump on his shoulder was significantly smaller and less painful. Cathy is continuing to offer Reiki to Sparky regularly, which is helping to mitigate his symptoms.

Lesson: No condition is too big for Reiki to help.

CASE HISTORY

Canine Teacher: Rugby

Reiki Practitioner: Kimberly Swan

Challenge: Eleven-year-old Australian shepherd suffers from a sore back.

Kimberly shares, "Smile is what Rugby does, with wide-mouthed, vocal kisses. Rugby is an 11-year-old Australian shepherd I first met four years ago. Before I met him, when he was a young agility star, he suffered from an injury that ended his career. At the time alternative therapies like massage and physiotherapy were not available,

TRY THIS
Healing Water Meditation

Sit comfortably and close your eyes. Imagine you are sitting in a beautiful Japanese garden next to a koi pond. Many beautiful and colorful koi reside just below the surface of the water near to you. Open yourself to connecting with the koi. Feel what it would be like to live so closely to the element of water. Imagine you can submerge yourself like a koi in the water, and with each in-breath, breathe water energy up through your roots. For several minutes, on each out-breath, expand this water energy from your heart into the universe around you. Feel the strength of the water filling your entire being and helping your heart expand outward in courage.

The water shows us how to be with our animals: gentle and still when we need to be, yet strong and flexible, too. Feel how connecting to the koi helps you to experience what it is to "be" water. Feel your whole being as it is showered with a peaceful strength. Feel water washing away fears and uncertainties and purifying and strengthening your energy. Relax your breath, and just sit in this beautiful element for 20 to 30 minutes. You can periodically revisit the in and out breath to assist your focus if needed.

and the veterinarians at the time did not have many options for injured back muscles. Rugby has had to live with a sore back since then, even too sore for massage at times.

"To my delight, he loves Reiki. It has taken several Reiki sessions, but Rugby is no longer too sore for massage. Mind you, it is still on his terms. Despite how sore Rugby was and how long he has been in pain, he never lets it show; he is always positive and happy. Greeting each day with a smile is some good advice."

Lesson: Reiki can help support healing, even in injuries that may have happened a long time ago.

CASE HISTORY

Canine Teacher: Rockie

Reiki Practitioner: Carol A. Hulse

Challenge: Nine-year-old Shih Tzu/Chihuahua mix has difficulty in navigating stairs due to a possible back problem.

When Carol arrived at Rockie's house, Rockie was lying on his bed a few feet from where she sat to offer Reiki. Carol remembers, "Rockie remained very relaxed throughout the treatment, yawning a few times. He snoozed a lot and intermittently opened his eyes to look directly at me. At one point, Rockie changed his position to get as close to me as he could. When I looked at Rockie's sweet face as he soaked up the Reiki, I felt that I was doing something truly meaningful with my life by offering Reiki to animals. This was a truly magical and life-affirming moment for me. And after 45 minutes, Rockie decided our session was over. Much to my surprise, he nimbly wiggled down from his bed and scampered away. Since his treatment, Rockie easily goes up and down the stairs without assistance."

Lesson: Both dog and practitioner can benefit from the connections experienced during Reiki treatments.

CASE HISTORY

Canine Teacher: Bo

Reiki Practitioner: Tina Clark

Challenge: Seven-pound miniature pinscher is diagnosed with cancer.

When her dog Bo was diagnosed with a malignant adrenal tumor in 2007, Tina made the decision to immediately have her tumor surgically removed. Tina remembers, "This unfortunate experience was actually the catalyst in my becoming a certified Reiki practitioner, as I felt a more organic healing approach would nicely complement any of the more mainstream forms of treatment. I began to incorporate this powerful healing modality as an adjunct by giving Bo daily sessions of Reiki. Her miraculous recovery and pristine post-op test results to date have continued to amaze and delight her doctors."

Lesson: Reiki can support postoperative healing and recovery.

CASE HISTORY

Canine Teacher: Bright Eyes

Reiki Practitioner: Judy Bullard

Challenge: A dog is hit by a car.

Judy's dog Bright Eyes got loose from the house one day. Suddenly, Judy heard car brakes screech outside: Bright Eyes had been hit. She was having a seizure when Judy approached. She gently picked her up and took her immediately to the vet. She offered Reiki for the entire drive. For the first 10 minutes of the drive, Bright Eyes was completely limp, but suddenly she jumped awake and sat up very startled. Thankfully, the vet determined that she seemed fine, except for a scratch on her nose, and told Judy to take her home and watch her carefully for the next couple of days. Judy offered her

Reiki most of that night and many times over the next several days. Bright Eyes never had seizures again and showed no other symptoms. She recovered completely and lived another 10 years.

Lesson: Reiki is very helpful in emergency situations.

CASE HISTORY

Canine Teacher: Take

Reiki Practitioner: Kamrin MacKnight

Challenge: Shiba Inu suffers a fibrocartilagenous embolism (FCE).

Take was diagnosed with an FCE and prescribed four to six weeks of complete crate rest. The vet said there was nothing else she could do and expected Take to make an 80 percent recovery. Kamrin offered Take Reiki and had a team of complementary therapists also offering flower essence, animal communication, Shamanism, and acupuncture. Amazingly, within three weeks, Take was recovered by 90 percent.

Kamrin shares, "He has continued to improve and is about 99 percent recovered. The neurologist and other vets were amazed at the extent of his recovery. Without the energy work, I truly doubt that he would have had such success, and probably wouldn't be able to enjoy his favorite activities, such as freestyle, tracking, and nosework. This experience has also opened the eyes of our training friends, some of whom are now using Reiki and flower essences for themselves."

Lesson: Reiki is a great complement to other holistic modalities, which, when used in combination with each other, can support a miraculous recovery.

CHAPTER 15

Healing the Past: Lessons in Kindness and Trust

Be kind whenever possible. It is always possible.

—Dalai Lama

For me, trust and kindness go hand in hand. We cannot build trust without kindness; we cannot be kind if we do not trust. Kindness and trust are the foundation on which the rehabilitation of shelter and sanctuary animals is built. Many of the animals there have mountains to climb to get over their abusive pasts.

Some of the issues that shelters and sanctuaries see on a daily basis are dogs who have been starved, neglected, chained outside, and had their collars grow into their necks; dogs who have been burned, poisoned, and beaten; small animals who have been injured from rough handling; animals so traumatized by humans that the whites of their eyes show with any attempt at physical touch. Working and volunteering in shelters and sanctuaries is angel's work, as is offering Reiki there. Courage is the armor all must wear.

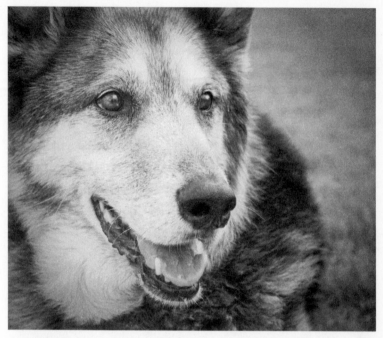

When we work or volunteer in shelters, we become aware of the darker side of humanity's treatment of animals. We learn of situations animals have faced that are so shocking they can shake us to our core. Some of my students tell me: "It's just too difficult for me. I can't go into that environment; it's too sad" (or depressing, or stressful—fill in the blank).

In the beginning, I felt that way, too. To give myself courage, I would look in the mirror before I went to offer Reiki in the shelter and say to myself, "If not you, then who will go?" I realized that my offer of Reiki may be the first kind experience that animal may have had in their lifetime. Maybe this could plant a seed of hope in that animal's heart, which could bloom with just a little tending. After witnessing so many shelter animals have wonderful responses to the Reiki treatments I offered, in time the memories of these positive healing experiences provided me with the bravery and determination I needed to keep going back.

As I've mentioned earlier, Reiki is not just about the energy itself; it's also about the person offering the energy. In other words, the dog is not just connecting with healing; he also is connecting with you as the facilitator. So your job is twofold: to create the space of healing for Reiki to do its work, and to create an experience of human interaction rooted in kindness, which (when coupled with the Reiki offered) can literally create miracles of healing.

In order to create that experience of loving connection for the dog, we must first courageously face the injustice of what the animal has experienced and, through the practice of compassion, release any other negative emotions that may overwhelm us when we think of the dog's past. Animals will be disturbed by emotions like fear, anger, and rage in us and may decide not to connect with us if we can't let go and approach them in a balanced, light state.

TRY THIS
Trust Affirmation

Sit with the word *trust* inside your heart and body for 3 to 5 minutes. Feel the meaning and truth of that word/emotion permeate your whole being. When you are ready, offer the word as a gentle, loving bridge of light from your heart to the heart of your animal. Include within the light all the feelings that go with the word. Continue holding that affirmation for an additional 3 to 5 minutes. Repeat as often as needed.

We reflect the dog's possibility to heal. In order to create a space of trust where the dog will connect with us—a space where anything can happen, including the dog being able to release and forgive the past—we also must able also release the past and find forgiveness in our own hearts. If we cannot do it ourselves, how can we expect the dog to do so? Dogs show us this so clearly. I began to see that the animals actually mirror for us what we need to do to help them: let go and forgive. In that moment of forgiveness, we experience compassion and kindness on a level so deep that anything in the realm of healing can happen!

In the early years, I frequently found that I had difficulty connecting with the animals who triggered the most emotion in me, often because I had just heard or read something terrible about their previous circumstances. I noticed that it was easier for me to stay calm as I sat with animals whose pasts I didn't know much about. The Reiki flowed easily, and the connection with the animal and healing responses seemed effortless.

I've learned that not knowing much, if anything, about the dog's health issues or problems can help me to stay in a positive space and allow the intuitive information to flow freely, without preconceived ideas or judgments. When I offer Reiki, I look for a place of emptiness inside myself—a place of letting go. Interestingly, I find that this is the place to which animals gravitate as well (sometimes on their own, and often with the assistance of Reiki). In this place, all of existence opens to the present moment, letting go of the past and not worrying about the future.

Many times over the years, I have heard people say, "This dog will not come near you," or "They won't come out of hiding while you are here." On the contrary, I have learned through Reiki that deep levels of trust are built very quickly, and that animals can often come right out of their shells, even if they've been there a long time. Offering Reiki with a gentle, light attitude is like bestowing a small kindness and then amping it up tenfold. Animals feel Reiki, sense its goodness, open to it, then come forward to thank us for it. It is as if, in being open to trusting us, they also begin to forgive their past human transgressors. As a result, we find ourselves assisting not only in healing the present but also in healing the very human/animal dynamic that has existed in that animal's previous experience.

Some animals simply and effortlessly embody the lesson of trust. One particular shelter dog's ability to live in trust and with forgiveness made quite an impression upon me. I had no knowledge of this dog's background or history. I was simply asked to work with an extremely playful and hyper young pit bull.

As he pranced and bounded around the treatment room, I wondered if he would ever decide to settle into the treatment and soak up the energy. After several minutes, he stopped his bouncing, walked slowly over to me, and sat down directly in front of me, leaning against my crossed legs. I put my hands on him, one hand on his chest, the other on his back, and just allowed the energy to flow. Soon he began to yawn, over and over. My hands felt very hot, and the space felt very peaceful.

TRY THIS
Willow and Wind Meditation

Imagine you are a beautiful weeping willow tree. Your branches spread out tall and wide, reaching all the way to the ground. Your roots carry you deep into the earth, making you stable and balanced. Imagine your dog is sitting next to you, to your weeping willow. You see that there is something from the

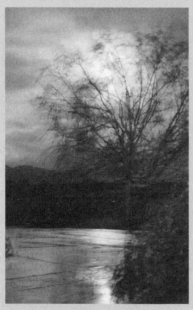

past that needs healing. Set your intention that you are open to facilitating healing for your dog in whatever way he is open to receive. Imagine a wind beginning to blow. Breathe in through your roots the energy of the earth. Breathe out into the wind. Feel your breath becoming one with the wind all around you. Imagine the air can heal and carry away anything your dog might be holding onto but ready to release.

Feel the wind blowing through your leaves. Feel your branches swaying to and fro. While staying stable in the earth, you can feel yourself becoming one with the wind. Feel its power to move and expand beyond the past and into a future of healing. See your dog as easily releasing any fears or worries from the past into the wind. See the wind picking up all those things needing to be healed in a swirling and powerful gust, blowing them away, where they dissipate in the healing energy of the universe. Hold this visualization for 20 to 30 minutes, revisiting the in and out breaths when needed for focus.

After about half an hour, he moved away and began to sniff the room's perimeters. It was clear that he was finished and ready to move onto other things. I called him over to me to thank him and give him a few scratches, and he bounded over joyfully, almost knocking me over in his enthusiasm. His whole body was wagging with gratitude. He was all love, happiness and sweetness. And in just being himself, he put a smile on my face: His joy was contagious!

Out of curiosity, I decided to ask the shelter staff person about his background. What I discovered was very different from what I had suspected. Apparently, a Good Samaritan had found this pit bull lying with another dog by the curb of a busy street. The other dog had already passed away, and this one was so weak he couldn't even lift his head. When he had first arrived at the shelter, three months previously, he had weighed only half of what he did now. Humans had clearly failed this dog in his past. But for him, the past was of no consequence. He was living in the moment, building upon the foundation of kindness the shelter had offered him during his three-month stay.

It was clear to me that this dog, through kindness and trust, was healing both his physical and emotional issues. His receptiveness to Reiki confirmed his openness to go deeper into his healing process. I felt sure he would find a family who could match his joy, and together they could amplify the happiness of all!

CASE HISTORY

Canine Teacher: Zeke

Reiki Practitioner: Mary Alice Santoro

Challenge: Seven-year-old rescued miniature schnauzer has nightmares.

Mary Alice adopted Zeke, a seven-year-old miniature schnauzer, along with his mother, who were both in an abusive home. Shortly after Mary Alice brought the dogs home, Zeke began to have nightmares. He would cry and sob frightfully in his sleep.

As Mary Alice remembers, "One afternoon, as he was sitting on my lap, I thought I'd give Reiki a try. I explained to him what Reiki was and asked permission to give him a treatment. I told him we would stop whenever he felt he had enough. Without thinking, I put my hands on him to start. He immediately turned around, gave me a strange look, jumped off my lap and ran from the room."

From then on, Mary Alice always started by offering Zeke Reiki from a distance—sometimes from across the room with me, and sometimes from an adjacent room. When Zeke was in another room and Mary Alice started offering him Reiki, he would eventually always wander into the room and lay down close to her. Over time, he began to show signs of improvement. His nightmares have significantly decreased in frequency and intensity. Mary Alice says, "Little by little, Zeke is learning to trust and learning to live without fear. I truly believe that Reiki can be the bridge between healing the emotional wounds of the past, resulting in a trusting and loving animal companion."

Lesson: Reiki is a great support to emotional healing.

CASE HISTORY

Canine Teacher: Tammy

Reiki Practitioner: Lynn Thiel

Challenge: Abused rescue dog shows intense fear of people.

Lynn adopted Tammy a few years ago from a local rescue group. Tammy had a terrible fear of people and would growl and show her teeth anytime Lynn got near her. At first, Lynn was very frightened of Tammy, then decided to offer her Reiki. After just a few minutes, Tammy began to calm down. Lynn offered Tammy Reiki every day, and over time she began to trust and accept Lynn. Lynn says, "This precious little dog made me such a better person. Thank you, Tammy, for the world."

Lesson: Reiki can support us in showing patience and kindness that can help even deep emotional wounds heal.

CHAPTER 16

Healing Anxiety-Related Behavior and Stress: Lessons in Finding Peace

See for yourself what brings you contentment, clarity, peace.
That is the path for you to follow.
   —The Buddha

When I first learned Reiki many years ago, my motivation was self-healing. I had learned of Reiki from my mom-in-law, Judy, after she experienced some amazing results healing from post-surgery complications. To humor her, I tried a treatment for myself. For me, Reiki felt like a massage times a thousand! I dropped almost immediately into an extremely relaxed state, totally free of stress, and my mind emptied of all concerns and worries for the entire treatment time. The hour treatment felt like five minutes. I was totally amazed! As I drove home, I knew I would have to learn this technique for myself.

Having struggled with anxiety problems from an early age, I instinctively knew from my very first experience with Reiki that it could heal me from the inside out. To be able to go so deeply and so easily into a state of deep relaxation was truly an amazing gift for a person like me. Over the years, working with Reiki, I have seen my problems with anxiety lessen—now they are few and far between, rather than a daily and overwhelming occurrence.

Probably because of my own personal experience with healing anxiety and stress in my own life, I have always felt a certain kinship and understanding with animals suffering from anxiety and stress-related problems, especially those in shelter environments. From the first days of my Reiki practice,

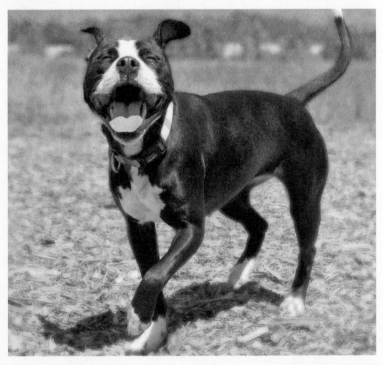

I began to volunteer in a local shelter, offering Reiki to the animals there. The shelter environment is probably one of the most stressful situations an animal can find itself in, and I can't think of a better place to bring Reiki!

I believe this so strongly, I co-founded a nonprofit organization to bring Reiki to shelters: Shelter Animal Reiki Association (SARA) with my friend Leah D'Ambrosio. The purpose of SARA is to bring standardized and professional, high-quality Reiki treatment and training programs to shelters and sanctuaries around the world. To date, SARA has more than 80 members across the United States, Canada, England, and Australia. The organizations belonging to SARA have experienced phenomenal results with their animals. Time and again we hear the staff saying, "Thank you for helping bring peace to our animals."

Many years ago, a shelter dog named Trooper experienced a profound healing of anxiety during a Reiki treatment with me. His story has always stayed with me, reminding me that there is no case that Reiki cannot help. I'll always remember the way he looked when I first saw him: his body low to the ground, slinking like a lizard rather than strutting like the powerful pit bull that he was. It was clear that he'd been abused or traumatized in the past.

I brought him to the inside office where I often gave treatments. All the way there, his body crouched no more than an inch or two off the ground. Every few steps he would stop suddenly in fear, as if he wasn't going to survive the short trip. Finally, we reached the quiet room where we could relax for Reiki.

I began the treatment by introducing myself to Trooper and letting him know that I was there to offer him Reiki, which would help him heal. I let him know that receiving the treatment was his choice. At first, he nervously wandered around the office. But after a few moments, he began to relax, choosing to push his body into my hands, sighing deeply, and resting his head on the floor. The office dog, a blind and deaf miniature poodle, came over and also pushed himself into my lap to absorb some Reiki as well. The atmosphere of the entire office became quiet, relaxed, and incredibly peaceful.

After about an hour of treatment, Trooper woke up, turned around to face me, and gave me that familiar look that many of my "Reiki dogs" give that means, "Thanks for the Reiki. I'm done now." I thanked Trooper for his openness to healing and took him back to his kennel. The difference in him was extraordinary. He was now walking normally, his body no longer slinking along the ground. He was also more responsive and less frightened of the world around him.

One of the staff immediately noticed his transformation and exclaimed, "He looks so much calmer than before!" This newfound calmness would later assist in his adoption. This is another reason why I love offering Reiki to anxious shelter animals: It is common for there to be almost immediate stress relief. No matter how stressed out or anxious the animals may initially be, Reiki can help them become calm and relaxed. It feels wonderful to witness the change in their behavior and a peaceful look in their eyes take the place of fear.

Because of the role of Reiki in my own life in healing anxiety, I felt especially humbled to have been able to assist

TRY THIS
Peace Affirmation

Close your eyes and sit comfortably with the word *peace* inside your heart and body for several minutes. Feel the meaning and truth of that word/emotion permeate your whole being. Imagine what it would look like if your animal were perfectly peaceful and calm. Hold that vision, as if it is already achieved, within your heart and mind for several minutes. When you are ready, offer the possibility of peace as a gentle, loving bridge of light, from your heart to the heart of your animal. Include within the light all the emotions that go with the word. Continue holding that affirmation and bridge of light for an additional several minutes.

Trooper's healing process. How beautiful to see that he was able to trust and connect with me and with Reiki, despite his difficult past. It's also a great lesson in how letting go of fear can open the door to new positive possibilities.

Immediate responses to Reiki do happen and are a wonderful testament to the power of the energy. But it's important to restate: We must not become attached to the outcome of the treatments. Response is not so immediate in some animals I've worked with over the years; healing requires patience and a dedication to offering regular Reiki treatments to the dog over a period of time. In the beginning, I found this frustrating. Why did this animal heal so quickly, while another one is taking so much time and patience? Eventually, I began to see that just as each animal has his own unique life experience and healing journey, the Reiki process will also look different for everyone.

TRY THIS
Healing Rock Meditation

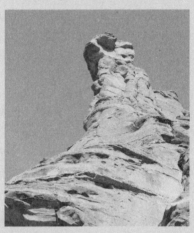

Sit comfortably with your dog. Close your eyes, and set your intention that you are open to facilitate healing for whatever your dog is open to receiving. Imagine you are a giant rock on the side of a craggy mountain, high up in the clouds. Place your hands so that they are palms down on your lap.

As you breathe in, imagine the breath moves from the earth, up your feet, spine, and hands, filling your whole body. On the out breath, imagine the breath returning down your body and back into the earth. With each breath, feel your strength, stability, and connection to the earth growing stronger. Your body begins to feel heavier and heavier. At the same time, your emotions begin to feel lighter and lighter. It is as if the closer you come to earth, the more peaceful your mind can become.

Once you have created this peaceful, rooted place within yourself, imagine that you can hold that space for your dog. Simply "invite" him into the space of your rock for healing. Within this space, there is perfect balance and calm. Hold this space for 20 to 30 minutes, revisiting the in and out breaths when needed for focus.

In letting go of our preconceived notions of "the healing timeline" for animals, and allowing them to heal in their own ways and at their own speed, we can begin to let go of our ego and become more open to the energy flow. Interestingly, our human ideas about what "should" be happening, or "how long" this or that will take to heal, may interfere with our ability to find peace within ourselves during treatments. We may find the voices within our heads chattering loudly at us: "Why?" "When?" "How?"

Imagine how an animal must feel, as we sit with them hoping that they will release anxiety while we ourselves are a ball of anxiety about the process! When we learn to relax and simply be present for the animal without judgment, we will find it is much easier to connect with animals, and in turn, we will begin to see better responses from them.

CASE HISTORY

Canine Teacher: Kaci

Reiki Practitioner: Leah D'Ambrosio

Challenge: Shelter dog is severely depressed.

Kaci's story began when she was brought to a shelter by a Good Samaritan after being tied to a tree for six years. The shelter staff worked with her for several months. She was finally adopted, but sadly returned a couple of months later. After six more months in the shelter, Kaci began to "crash," a phenomenon all too common in shelter dogs. She no longer wanted to eat, howled for hours after closing time, and became deeply depressed. Leah had just completed her volunteer training for special needs dogs and asked if she could work with Kaci.

Leah remembers, "Our first meeting was difficult, as all Kaci wanted to do was climb in my lap. After a few minutes of me reassuring her I wouldn't leave and that I was going to offer Reiki, she laid calmly half in my lap and half on the floor. She was so needy, she couldn't stand not to touch me. As the Reiki started flowing, her body relaxed and her breathing slowed down. Although she never closed her eyes, she ended the treatment more relaxed than I had seen her in a very long time.

"The second week, we started our session with her laying next to me and her paw laid gently on my open hand. We sat together in this beautiful Reiki space for 30 minutes or so, when a couple came by to look at the information on her door. Kaci glanced up but quickly closed her eyes and went back into her space. I felt the sadness and hopelessness flow out of her. She had been disappointed so many times by people, she had finally given up. As we sat there, I whispered to her that she had the power to pick the people she wanted and that she did not have to wait for someone to pick her. She kept her eyes closed and acted like she didn't hear me, so I stopped and kept the Reiki flowing. The couple finally left, and Kaci and I both sighed.

"We had been sitting in the Reiki space for about 10 minutes since the couple had left when a staffer came in to tell us that Kaci was wanted up front by some potential adopters. I told them we were finished and whispered again to Kaci that she can choose her family. Off she went to the front of the shelter, and I went to log out and end my day. "As I was leaving the shelter I had to pass Kaci, her potential adopters, and a couple of shelter staff who were discussing her needs and requirements. I started walking to the side of them so I wouldn't interrupt, when Kaci suddenly jumped in front of me with a big doggy smile on her face and her tail wagging frantically. As clear as if someone had said it out loud, I heard, 'I found them! I found my new family!' It was nothing short of a miracle.

"The next day I went to the shelter wishing I would not see her, and luckily my wish came true. I was told she was adopted by a lovely couple who had Akita experience and felt they had found the perfect dog in Kaci."

Lesson: Reiki can help the true spirit of a dog come out, making it easier for potential adopters to connect.

CASE HISTORY

Canine Teacher: Marlie

Reiki Practitioner: Allison Culver

Challenge: Yellow Lab rescued from a puppy mill seeks emotional healing.

Marlie was rescued from her life as a breeding dog for a puppy mill and adopted into a loving family. She had many physical challenges that set her back, including a stomach perforation, fungal infections, and ongoing joint issues, but her most urgent need was emotional. Marlie's adopter, Cindy, noticed that Marlie would not socialize with others, seemed sad and depressed, and kept herself isolated in her crate all day long.

As Allison offered Reiki to Marlie, the dog's body shook as she moaned and groaned. Finally, she let out the loudest, longest moan Allison had ever heard. After this moan of release, the change in Marlie was immediate! She began wagging her tail, bouncing like a puppy, and asking to be petted! She began to play with her canine sibling and take walks enthusiastically. Marlie's person, Cindy, says, "Never could I have believed the change that would occur with just one session. It has impacted not just Marlie's life but the lives of all of us who have come to know the true spirit that is Marlie."

Lesson: Reiki can help dogs release emotional issues from their past.

CASE HISTORY

Canine Teacher: Ida

Reiki Practitioner: Ann Noyce

Challenge: Retired racing greyhound has severe fear of thunderstorms.

Ann offered Reiki several times to support Ida's emotional healing. She remembers one treatment, in particular, when Ida quickly settled down with her back snuggled in Ann's hands. The dog was very relaxed and beginning to fall asleep. A small thunderstorm began rumbling through the area. Almost immediately, Ida lifted her head and started panting, and her body began to noticeably tremble, yet she remained lying down with her back resting against Ann's hands. As it rained and rumbled, Ida just lay there panting and trembling with the thunder.

Ann shares, "As we sat there in the Reiki space, Ida slowly began to calm down. The panting stopped, and I could feel the trembling become less and less, until Ida fell into a deep Reiki nap. We shared this beautiful quiet time during the thunderstorm for another 10 to 15 minutes or so. Ida remained in a very deep sleep as I thanked her and quietly left."

Since this series of treatments, Ida's mom reports that whenever there is a thunderstorm, Ida will bark to acknowledge it and then go back to doing whatever she is doing. She no longer pants, trembles, or paces for the duration of the thunderstorm.

Lesson: Reiki can help animals release fear.

CHAPTER 17

Healing from Loss: Lessons in Love and Compassion

Two strays seeking warmth
A dog and I in the sun
Sharing Loneliness.
   —Cliff Edwards

Some of the most difficult issues we deal with in life, whether we are dogs or humans, are issues surrounding loss—loss of physical abilities, loss of an important emotional relationship, loss of a physical place to live. In my experience, the process of healing involves filling the space left by loss with love.

So much of my journey with animals has been one of the heart. My heart's purpose on this earth is to share the love I feel for animal-kind. I have seen animals healed through human love, humans healed through the love of their animals, and animals and humans healing each other in love and compassion. Reiki seems to offer me a special lens through which I view the world, one where I can see the spirits and hearts of beings, not just their physical struggles. Through the Reiki connection, my awareness has somehow been amplified and focused, and I have seen extraordinary things happen.

I have assisted many animals, as well as my human students, in using Reiki to heal the issues that are left behind when there is loss. As a result, I have become much more aware of the power of the love that we humans have for our animals, and the love and compassion our animals give us in return, as well as to each other.

There is an unfortunate species-ism among humans, often resulting from our cultural conditioning. We see it, for

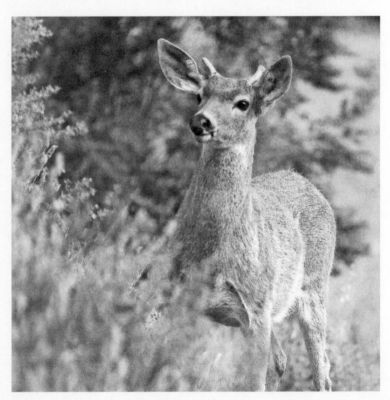

example, in judgments that humans make about the comparative worth of animals in a world dominated by man, using statements like, "This is a superior human; that is just a lowly animal." From where I sit, it's clear to me that humans are not the only beings with the ability to live from the heart and radiate compassion.

The story I would like to share in this chapter involves my dog only tangentially and is primarily about an experience with a deer. I have included it here because it is one of my most memorable Reiki experiences.

One October evening, my husband and I were out driving and encountered a horrific scene: a beautiful young buck with two-inch horns run over by an SUV just as we drove past. I offered the deer Reiki and felt an immediate heat and *whoosh* of white light flooding through my body as well as a sense of peace and understanding from the deer. I sensed that the deer's spirit had lingered on the street, not realizing he had passed, but the Reiki had allowed him to be carried gently and surely into the light.

Although I knew Reiki had helped this deer, I felt overwhelmed by the difficult reality faced by deer living in the midst of human civilization. I could not erase the image of carnage from my mind. I wondered if I'd ever be able to sleep again without nightmares.

Later that night, I took my dear dog Dakota for his evening stroll. As we walked outside, I could hardly believe my eyes: Standing in silent vigil across the street from my home was another buck. It looked just like the one I had seen earlier in the evening, with identical two-inch horns. Although we had lived in that house for four years, we had never seen a deer in our neighborhood. Had I not come outside to walk my dog, I would have missed this scene entirely.

I stood still, awestruck by his gaze. We stared at each other for a long time, and it dawned on me that he was a messenger, come to say, "Have courage and hope." As soon as this thought crossed my mind, the buck turned away and walked slowly away into the dark night, his form eventually being swallowed by the mist. That night I slept peacefully, with the image of the healthy young deer in my mind.

A few months later, a student of mine asked me to offer Reiki to a fawn whose mother had been hit and killed by the side of the highway. Wildlife volunteers and animal control were unable to catch the fawn, and he refused to leave his mother's body. Everyone worried for the fawn's safety by the highway, his weakened state without his mother's milk, and feared a negative outcome.

At that time, I had a baby of my own at home who was still nursing, so I felt a special personal connection to this situation. Rather than descend into worry, though, I remembered the two young bucks I had encountered a few months previously, and the message of hope they had imparted. As I began to offer Reiki to the doe who had passed away, as well as her fawn, I just knew that the perfect solution would be found (although I couldn't imagine what that could be). Courage and hope—those were the words I kept telling myself.

A few days later, my student contacted me with unbelievable news: Two young bucks had arrived out of nowhere, adopted the fawn, and taken her with them. The experts were

TRY THIS
Rainbow Heart Connection

Sit quietly for several minutes and connect to the energy of your heart. Breathe in air from the earth into your heart. Visualize your heart as a beautiful center of white light within your being. Imagine this light is filled with all the love and compassion you have experienced in your lifetime. On your out breath, see this light, with all the colors of a rainbow, expanding from your heart, beyond your physical body, into your aura, the room, and out into the universe.

Next, bring to mind an animal in your life that you would like to connect with for healing in love and compassion. See the energy of the animal's heart as a beautiful center of white light within his or her being. Expand the rainbow of your heart in love, compassion, serenity, and peace to include the heart of your dog. Remembering that this light is merely an "offering" on your part, and that if the animal is willing your hearts can unify in a beautiful space of healing through this rainbow.

Spiritually, rainbows symbolize hope, harmony, and connection beyond the physical. Visualize your hearts unified in rainbow light and perfectly in balance, at peace, connected, and completely healed. Know that there is no situation that cannot be healed, that there is always hope, and that you will always be connected to each other, no matter what. Hold this image in your mind for 20 to 30 minutes, revisiting the visualization of in and out breaths when needed for focus.

amazed, as this was highly unusual, but they believed that with the help of the two bucks, the fawn would be able to survive. Already anticipating the answer, I asked my student to describe the bucks. Sure enough, one of them had two-inch horns.

Even as I relate this story to you now—and it has been almost five years since this event occurred—I still feel awestruck by the outcome. I cannot explain how all these connections occurred, except to say that animals are energetically wise beyond our understanding. I know that they feel their connection to each other in a much more fundamental way than we humans do. Perhaps this is one of the reasons they are so receptive to Reiki—we are finally speaking a language that is familiar to them. I can also say with certainty that animals know about loss, but they also know about the healing power of love and compassion. I also believe that through our intention to connect with them energetically, we are truly changed and our awareness deepens.

CASE HISTORY

Canine Teachers: Jake and Bailey

Reiki Practitioner: Linda Frampton

Challenge: Rescued German shepherd misses his canine companion.

When Jake became ill with kidney problems, Linda was able to offer Reiki on his last day. Jake's person, Jai, noted how much more peaceful he became after the treatment. After his passing, Linda again offered Reiki. She recalls, "I visualized him rolling on his back in the grass and suddenly felt very happy. I smelled the beautiful perfume of honeysuckle and felt that Jake was saying thank you to Jai for letting him go and that he was now happy, pain free, and in a peaceful place."

Jai confirmed that Jake used to roll on his back in this fashion when he was happy and that (unbeknownst to Linda) they had honeysuckle growing in their garden along the fence where Jake used to play. Jai felt much better knowing that they had made the right decision to help him on his way, and that he was indeed grateful.

Linda remembers, "After a few days, Jai told me that Bailey was obviously missing Jake and that he was still very quiet and not quite himself. So I went to their house to offer some Reiki to Bailey. He came to sit beside me on the floor and lay out alongside my leg to receive some hands-on healing. I tried to relay the information to him that Jake was in a peaceful place and happy now, but would not be coming back to Bailey in his physical form, although his spirit would still be around Bailey if he needed him. When Bailey had received enough Reiki, he got up and went to lie in the place where Jake always used to lay down in the living room. Until that point, Bailey had not been anywhere near Jake's special place since his passing. After the healing, Bailey seemed to accept that Jake had gone and was able to move on with his life."

Lesson: Reiki is helpful before, during, and after a dog's transition. It can bring comfort and healing to the whole family.

CHAPTER 18

Healing in Transitions: Lessons in Hope

In my mind I walk
With you along the ocean
Waves licking my feet
  —Judy Prasad

This haiku was written by my mother-in-law to honor the passing of my beloved dog, Dakota, who was in many ways the heart of our family for 16 years. As I began this book, I wondered how I would write this chapter. I knew it was coming, but I waited a long time to write it. How could I put into words the experience of caring for my dearest Dakota through hospice and transition?

Now that I stand on the other side of this most difficult journey, I am here to tell those of you walking this road with your animals that Reiki allows you to hold them, support them, and create peace for them right up until the very end—and even beyond. I promise you: You can do it. Reiki will help you find your courage. It is there, inside you—all the strength you need to get through this, gracefully and harmoniously.

Still, preparing for the physical separation can be very difficult and dark at times. I find this quote from Aikido master and founder Morihei Ueshiba of particular comfort:

Loyalty and devotion lead to bravery.
Bravery leads to the spirit of self-sacrifice.
The spirit of self-sacrifice creates trust in the power of love.

As your animals have been devoted to you throughout their lives, so will you now devote yourself to supporting the final chapter in their life journeys. It will not be easy: You will have to muster all the courage you have inside. You will find sleep and rest hard to come by—sometimes nonexistent—but you will forge ahead because of the love that encompasses your heart. This love—which is really just the energy of your heart—is what will get you through the difficult journey of holding your animals' paws in your hands as they cross to the other side.

My own journey of supporting the transition of my dearest dog, Dakota, began in March 2008, when he was diagnosed with cancer in the bladder and lungs. My initial reaction was of disbelief and shock, followed by an overwhelming sense of helplessness and sadness. I then went into "Reiki mode" and realized I could offer Reiki to Dakota every day. This empowered me, giving me purpose and hope. I had seen many miracles with Reiki healing over the years, and after all, as this is my calling, I felt sure that Reiki could "cure" Dakota, if I worked hard enough. So I hoped. How much I had still to learn.

The first lesson Dakota taught me was to remember to begin with my own self-healing. I am sure that animals do not fear death, but they do fear for us, our emotions, and our worry. Dakota had been my constant companion and protector for many years. We were so closely bonded, I knew he was feeling every part of my worry and sadness.

The first night after Dakota's diagnosis, as I sat with him to offer Reiki, he turned away and said "no." I was shocked! "But Dakota," I pleaded with him, "This is what I do. I know I can cure you. Please let me do Reiki with you!" In my earnestness and emotion, my ego had taken over. Again he pulled away, agitated. And so, as I so often instruct my students, I realized I must respect his wishes and went to bed, not sure of how to proceed.

The next evening's session proceeded in the same manner. This time, however, I was nearly hysterical about it. "Dakota, why won't you let me do Reiki with you?" Out of habit from my self-healing practice, as my anxiety rose, I put my hands over my heart and offered Reiki to myself for calm and peace. Dakota looked at me then—really looked at me. As our eyes met, I knew that, at that moment, he desperately wanted me to do Reiki for myself—not for him, but for myself. "I'm fine," he seemed to say. "You need this!"

And so I did as he wished: Instead of offering him Reiki, I began my own Reiki meditation. About five minutes into the meditation, he stopped watching me, lay his head down, let out a huge sigh, and went to sleep. By the end of my 30-minute meditation, he was snoring peacefully. As I took a deep breath and came out of my meditation, I looked at him and realized that he, too, had received healing.

So the most basic lesson that Dakota taught me, as we began his long journey into spirit, was to go back to the beginning and take care of myself first. I had to be in a peaceful place before I could offer him anything. The peace and calm that radiates within us will be a healing balm for our animals. We are already so connected to them. When we create change in our own inner space, they will be also changed. As we nurture our inner peace, they also will be uplifted and comforted.

Dakota benefited from a combination of allopathic drugs, acupuncture, Chinese herbs, and sharing my daily Reiki meditations. As the weeks of care turned into months, we had many positive physical results. His bladder tumors shrank to almost nothing (and one of them even disappeared), so that he could control his bladder and urinate without discomfort. The pain medications he was on for the lung tumors usually tear up the stomach, but he was eating regularly and still looking forward to every meal and treat; his digestion was completely normal. (He never had even one bout of diarrhea.)

My one-year-old daughter, Indigo, began to notice that Dakota was becoming less mobile, falling often. She would carefully save a few of her Cheerios at snack time and walk over to him, dropping them near his front feet so that he could reach them. Dakota began to watch Indigo and beg for a treat every time she had food. The way he would crane his neck and tilt his head, giving her his "cute face" so that she would notice him, was a sight to behold! And she never disappointed him. She would always have a bite or two to share, and would giggle endlessly as he tried to catch the falling crumbs. For

Indigo and Dakota, there were only lightness and joy in these innocent and precious moments, and I longed to bask in that space with them.

Still, I began to accept the inevitable. Dakota's hind legs stopped working, but he was too weak to use a sling or wheelchair. He was soon unable even to turn over. Because of the tumors in his lung, he was no longer able to lie on his left side. I had to pick him up and carry him out to do his business in the yard because he refused, in all his dignity and pride, to "mess" in the house.

Carrying a 45-pound dog in and out of the house several times a day and at night began to take its toll on my back, not to mention my sleep. As I somehow carried on, moving through each 24-hour period, caring for Dakota as well as my one-year-old daughter, I realized the truth of Gail Pope's (of BrightHaven) words: that each and every day, Dakota was teaching me lessons in "love, acceptance, joy, courage, and fearlessness."

Each night, I continued with the Reiki meditation, with me sitting next to Dakota doing Reiki for myself and not focusing on him, and him relaxed and sleeping each time. I could feel on a very deep level that we were growing closer and closer to transition. Then one morning around 5 a.m., a few days before he died, I took him out to pee in the front yard. It was very hard for him to stand on his front feet, and my back was beginning to give out from the weeks of carrying him in and out every few hours 24/7. I felt so hopeless and alone at that moment and very, very sad.

Suddenly, I felt someone watching me and looked up. On the hill across the street I saw the dark outline of a doe staring intently at us. (I should mention that we had moved to a new town and no longer resided at the home where we had formerly seen the deer with the two-inch horns across the street.)

The sky had just begun to show the pink of sunrise behind her, and I could see her perfect form in the light. It was the most peaceful, beautiful nature scene—like something out of *National Geographic*. The feeling of the doe's calm grace felt like a blessing and balm upon my saddened heart. She stayed there for the 15 minutes or so that we were outside, watching

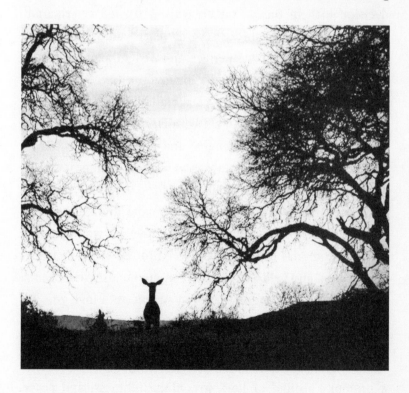

me first holding Dakota, then setting him down for a bit, then carrying him back inside. I can't describe how it comforted me to feel her presence that whole time. Truly, it was a healing for both Dakota and me.

We often think of animals seeking us out when they are in need of healing. But sometimes—especially for those of us who spend so much time in the inner intention of helping animals—well, sometimes, I believe, they come to help *us*. We really help each other, when all is said and done. How wonderful that I would receive such a timely healing visit from this doe.

On July 5, 2008, my husband and I made the difficult decision to help Dakota on his way. A trusted veterinarian, who had known Dakota for several years, came to our home that day. The weather was perfect, and we let Dakota spend the morning out on the lawn under his favorite tree. After a final meal, which he ate with gusto, Dakota lay down one last time with us. My husband and I sat with Dakota and talked about our best moments, trips, laughs, and memories from our 16 years living together. Dakota was so relaxed, so at peace, more so than I could remember him being for a very long time.

When the veterinarian arrived, Dakota greeted him, and I felt that he knew very clearly why the vet was there; he seemed grateful. I began to offer Reiki for all of us, there under the tree, and held Dakota's face in my hands. We looked at each other as I whispered, "I love you. Let go. I love you. It's okay to let go. Let go, sweetheart, let go."

And at the moment he passed. I felt the energy of his spirit lift out of his body and encompass my heart. It was such a profound feeling of love, joy, bliss, lightness, and peace, such as I had never known. It lasted just a moment, then I felt only stillness. What a gift to be able to connect with him as he had passed.

I truly believe that, as Rita Reynolds has said in her wonderful book, *Blessing the Bridge*, "Once a connection of souls is consciously made, the link is eternal and unlimited. I am sure we will meet again. A bond of love always forms a thread between us and our animal companions that can never be broken."

As I write these words, tears still flow freely from me. Perhaps they always will when I revisit that day. I cannot begin to express the gifts of love, lessons, and light that Dakota, my very first animal Reiki teacher, bestowed upon my life. Here it is, more than four years later, and still I dedicate my meditation practice each night to him. He is the inspiration for Shelter Animal Reiki Association (SARA), my nonprofit organization, which I have officially dedicated to him. I still feel him sitting at my feet in all the classes that I teach. He is still with me so strongly in spirit, motivating me, guiding me, and protecting me, I believe.

It has taken some time for me to be able to write about this experience. At first, the gifts and lessons learned throughout my final months with Dakota were obscured in a haze of emotion. But in time, as healing of my heart continued and I walked farther along the road of darkness, grief, and separation, I found myself drawn to the light of compassion and love—this is his legacy, and in this place we will never be separated. I urge each of you reading this book who is walking this road of transition with your animal to take heart—remember that your energy will always be one. The outer layer only will be separated, but on the deepest level, you will always be connected. As Rita Reynolds writes in *Blessing the Bridge*:

> When I hold a dying creature either in my arms or in my mind, I feel a merging of greater purpose that springs from Spirit, which is our true nature. When I do this, I believe it is the quintessence of compassion—the giving over of oneself directly into the needs, the calling out for help from another. It is the equivalent of being an angelic presence in human form, just as my animal friend is angel in animal form.

Dakota is one of many animals that I have worked with through transition, but because he was the closest to my heart, it was the most difficult. I have learned a deeper compassion and understanding for hospice workers and caregivers. I understand very clearly that the road to healing is not always an easy one. But despite the fact that this is our hardest work, in being present with animals who are passing on, our offering of Reiki brings many gifts.

First and foremost, it brings the gift of peace to the animal as the body dies, as well as to the humans who are grieving the physical loss. Second, it takes away the feeling of helplessness we feel when all other healing methods have run their course: With Reiki we can actually support the animal's transition out of the physical body and into spirit. Third, when we are in that Reiki meditative space, we begin to understand that the sense of separation we feel between life and death is

TRY THIS
Gratitude Affirmation

Sit with the words "I feel gratitude; each day is a precious gift" inside your heart and body for several minutes. Feel the meaning and truth of those words/emotions permeating your whole being. Think about all the experiences you've had with your animal for which you are grateful, all the parts of his or her unique being for which you are thankful. When you are ready, offer gratitude as a gentle, loving bridge of light from your heart to the heart of your animal. Include within the light all the feelings that go with the word. Imagine that the light can spread out to the hearts of all your family members and even encompass the whole home. Continue holding this affirmation for several more minutes.

simply a veil of perception. This awareness can help heal our understanding of our own death and the death of loved ones, both animal and human. We realize that death is not an ending; it's merely the beginning of a new chapter in the energetic journey of the spirit.

Recently, my sister called to tell me of a vivid and unusual dream she had had about us and Dakota. This is what I like to call a "Reiki dream," a dream that helps us go deeper into the layers of energetic existence.

In the dream, she and I were walking through the forest with a Native American shaman. The shaman was telling the story of my life with Dakota and all the gifts he had brought me. Suddenly, in the dream, there was a loud chiming of bells, as if from a cathedral, even though here we were in the middle of the woods.

"Do you hear that?" the shaman exclaimed. "Those are angels' bells. They ring every time an animal you have lost connects with you and knows that you are thinking about him. Dakota hears you. Never forget, he is still with us."

What a beautiful dream, and a wonderful metaphor to describe the energetic connection that remains strong in our hearts with the ones we love. Listen with your heart, and I know you will hear the bells of the dogs that you miss ringing loud and clear. Yes, truly, they are still here with you.

CASE HISTORY

Canine Teacher: Seamus

Reiki Practitioner: Colette Anusewicz

Challenge: Dog is diagnosed with advanced bone cancer.

After offering several Reiki treatments to Seamus, Colette received wonderful feedback from Paul, Seamus's person. He said, "We have not had to carry him around as much, and his mood has definitely changed. A week ago, he wouldn't get out of his bed. Now he looks forward to walks and is wagging his tail again."

Two months later, Colette was able to offer Reiki during Seamus's transition. She recalls her intense experience: "I felt an energy shift in my body, then I was totally immersed with an overwhelming powerful love. I could feel him leave his body, and he was now floating . . . it was very peaceful and he was surrounded with an intense love." Being able to offer Reiki to Seamus during the last two months of his life was very comforting to his person, Paul. He believes Reiki had a profound impact on how Seamus experienced these last two months.

Lesson: Reiki can support physical comfort in the days leading up to transition and can help support a peaceful transition. Practitioners can often connect to the transitional process on a very deep level through Reiki.

CASE HISTORY

Canine Teacher: Lucca

Reiki Practitioner: Michele Rodriguez

Challenge: Doberman pinscher is diagnosed with heart problems.

Michele received a call that Lucca was doing very poorly and on the path to passing. She remembers that she arrived "to find Lucca very despondent, very sad, and with eyes that had very little life in them. He could barely lift his head to greet me. Lucca's damaged heart was giving out, and all of his medicines were no longer working. I began Reiki on him while he lay in his bed." The next day he woke up and wanted to go outside to see his favorite rabbits, and he began to play with his little sister, Luna, for a brief time. Michele continued to offer him Reiki for the next four days, and by the end of the fourth day there had been some great changes in him.

Michele remembers, "He began to eat better, and the family noticed he was not laying in his bed so much. Before this, because of his weak heart, he never wanted to be active much, let alone play. Lucca greeted me at the car on my next visit. It was almost as if he was saying, 'You have saved my life.' He would find his favorite lounge chair in the backyard and climb up on it and receive his Reiki with the sun shining down on us. Over the next month he would get his strength back and his appetite. Even his medicine was decreasing, which the veterinarian could not believe. He was getting stronger and his eyes were beautiful and full of life again. It was as if Reiki had given him a new lease on life."

Michele continued Reiki once a week, then once a month, for the next couple of months. His body was transforming, taking on a different shape—even his muscular build was coming back. He began to be his old self again. He chased the rabbits again. He enjoyed running with his sister and taking walks and playing again.

After seven good months, Lucca began to have trouble breathing. One morning, he went out for his usual time in the backyard and decided to run and play with Luna. Instead, he collapsed in his favorite place in the yard and passed away. Michele says, "I'm honored and touched to have been his student."

Lesson: Reiki can improve quality of life, even for chronic conditions.

CHAPTER 19

Final Thoughts About Animals and Healing

The journey of a thousand miles begins with one step.
—Lao Tzu

My experience with Dakota through his last days and final journey into spirit was not only an ending but also a return to the beginning. I had begun my animal Reiki journey with him sitting atop my feet as I gave myself a Reiki treatment, and I ended our Reiki relationship in this life with the same focus inward—offering myself Reiki for those several months of hospice as he lay relaxed at my side.

Perhaps this is the greatest lesson the animals are pointing us toward: Healing begins inside each of us and moves outward naturally. It is nothing we can force or push upon another individual. The healing of the animals that we Reiki practitioners facilitate is simply a byproduct of the miracle that is healing energy. How surprising and unexpected!

This book got its start from my deep desire to share how Reiki can heal dogs, how you can "rescue" your dogs with Reiki. And indeed, I believe you can. Still, after 13 years of doing Reiki with animals, the healing energy has brought me back to myself—Reiki and the animals have also rescued *me*; in the shared space of Reiki connectedness, the animals have healed *me*. I have been changed, deepened, and made a better person simply by sharing the animals' energetic space and presence. Reiki has become more than a system of practice for me; it has become a way of life, a way of remaining mindful and trying to always be present, open, and connected.

I've read about people who go to India, Tibet, and other pilgrimage spots across the world in order to visit a holy temple or study with a guru. I've met people who've been "touched" by an enlightened being on this planet and have been forever changed by it. Well, I, too, have been touched by a beautiful light, a shining star of healing and compassion. It has shone upon me in the unlikeliest of forms—an abandoned guinea pig, a feral cat, an abused dog. I have seen the light shine from the eyes of a baby alligator, a wise raven, and a majestic lion. I have felt the presence of the light in the soft

TRY THIS
Opening to Possibilities

Sit in a relaxed posture with your eyes closed, breathing gently. With your mind, open your awareness to the "animal need" around you. Visualize yourself as you go through your day; see yourself as present, aware, and available to be a healing support in all that you do, everywhere you go, and for any animal that may choose to find you. Hold this focus for 5 to 10 minutes. This is a great exercise to start your day.

breath of a horse, the profound call of a whale, the vibrating footsteps of an elephant.

Many people may ask, "What can animals teach us? After all, we are human beings, and our brains are more evolved."

Well, I say that it's not about the evolution of the mind; it's about the evolution of the spirit. It's about our connection to energy, to animals, to our earth, to all of it—earth and sky, the yin and the yang, the two halves of the whole of existence. In the end, Reiki is really about our awareness of the interdependence of all things, our ability to live in the present moment, to forgive the past, and to accept with grace and dignity all things that cross our paths.

Through my experiences doing Reiki healing with dogs, I've come to realize that, actually, dogs are much more evolved than we are. The stories shared in this book—not only my own personal stories but also the stories contributed by other canine Reiki practitioners—show us that when we human beings open our hearts and minds to the dogs in our lives, the possibilities are infinite.

If we can let go of our human preconception that our species—humankind—is somehow superior to all other species, we can open to the infinite. With the practice of Reiki, we can learn to open our hearts. In this open and interconnected space of the infinite, we can learn the lessons of the animals—lessons in courage, forgiveness, compassion, love, and hope. And if we can nurture mindfulness and try to live in the space of compassionate intention every moment of every day, then perhaps our planet can someday find harmony and peace.

Whether we realize it or not, our journey on this earth begins with the animals and will end with the animals. I hope that the exercises, stories, and suggestions shared in this book have helped open the door to the possibility of connection inside your spirit. Go now. Share this goodness and light with the dogs that cross your path. I promise you that once they feel your openness to them, they will come forward as eager teachers. You have only to sit, breathe, listen, and open your heart.

Appendix

List of "Try This" Exercises

Resources

Animal Reiki

Organizations, Groups, and Websites

Animal Reiki Source

www.animalreikisource.com

Kathleen's teaching website. This is a resource for animal Reiki information, articles, worldwide practitioner directory, and a variety of audio, correspondence, telephone, and in-person courses.

Animal Reiki Source Yahoo Group

pets.groups.yahoo.com/group/animalreikisource

Kathleen created this group with the intention to support, connect, and network with the Animal Reiki community around the world. Members also offer free distant healing to animals in need.

The Animal Reiki Talk

www.animalreikisource.com/reiki-classes/animal-reiki-talk

The first Tuesday of each month, Kathleen offers this free teleclass. It is a time for animal Reiki practitioners to come together, connect and share stories, hear the wonderful animal Reiki work going on around the world, support each other, and ask questions. It is also a time for people interested in learning more about Animal Reiki to join in and listen.

Shelter Animal Reiki Association (SARA)
www.shelteranimalreikiassociation.org

SARA is a 501(c)3 nonprofit organization co-founded by Kathleen Prasad and Leah D'Ambrosio. Its purpose is to support through Reiki treatments and training: the growing number of Reiki practitioners who wish to establish programs in their local shelters, sanctuaries, and rescues; the animals and staff of those organizations; and the people and animals of the community at large. You can join SARA as a supporter now—just visit our website. We appreciate your support.

Publications

The Animal Reiki Handbook. Kathleen Prasad and SARA
  Members. San Rafael, CA: Shelter Animal Reiki
  Association, 2009.

If you are a Reiki practitioner hoping to reach out to a shelter, sanctuary, or rescue organization in your area, this book is for you!

Animal Reiki: Using Energy to Heal the Animals in Your
  Life. Kathleen Prasad and Elizabeth Fulton. Berkeley,
  CA: Ulysses Press, 2006.

A great introduction to Reiki for animals. Includes many wonderful real-life stories of animal healing.

These following books are collections of case studies from animal Reiki practitioners around the world. Included are many stories of the transformational power of Reiki in the lives of many species of animals. Available from lulu.com and Amazon:

Tails from the Source: Volume 1, 2001–2005: The Animal Reiki Resource Newsletter Collection. Kathleen Prasad, ed. lulu.com, 2011.

Animal Reiki Tails: Volume II. The Animal Reiki Resource Newsletter Collection. Kathleen Prasad, ed. lulu.com, 2011.

Animal Reiki Tails: Volume III. The Animal Reiki Resource Newsletter Collection. Kathleen Prasad, ed. lulu.com, 2011.

Reiki

Organizations, Groups, and Websites

The International House of Reiki

www.ihreiki.com

Kathleen recommends that all her students study with Frans Stiene of the International House of Reiki. She says, "The traditional Japanese approach of Reiki as a path of spiritual development is a profound energetic foundation that will help you immensely when you are working with animals."

Shibumi International Reiki Association

www.shibumireiki.org

A nonprofit professional international Reiki group that supports and promotes the Japanese art of the system of Reiki.

Publications

The Japanese Art of Reiki. Bronwen and Frans Stiene. Brooklyn, NY: O Books, 2005.

Detailed and structured meditative Reiki techniques with a martial arts bent.

The Reiki News Magazine. www.reiki.org.

Published by the International Center for Reiki training, this 80-page full-color glossy magazine contains articles on every aspect of Reiki practice written by Reiki practitioners from diverse backgrounds.

The Reiki Sourcebook, Revised and Expanded. Bronwen and Frans Stiene. Brooklyn, NY: O Books, 2009.

The "Reiki Bible." It gives a thorough account of all aspects of Reiki practice in the world today.

Reiki Techniques Card Deck. Bronwen and Frans Stiene. Brooklyn, NY: O Books, 2006.

A fun and intuitive way to treat yourself.

Your Reiki Treatment. Bronwen and Frans Stiene. Brooklyn, NY: O Books, 2007.

A detailed look at the Reiki treatment from the perspectives of both practitioner and client. Very thorough!

CDs

Order through www.ihreiki.com/shop:

Reiki Tenohira. Frans and Bronwen Stiene. International House of Reiki.

Guided practice of hand positions for self-treatment with meditation music.

Reiki Ho. Frans and Bronwen Stiene. International House of Reiki.

Guided practice of the traditional Japanese technique of Hatsurei Ho with meditation music.

Order through Amazon.com:

Reiki Meditations for Self-Healing: Traditional Japanese Practices for Your Energy and Vitality. Bronwen Stiene. Sounds True, 2008.

This CD offers guided instruction in traditional Japanese practices for your own health and vitality. Requiring no prior experience in the system, this program guides listeners through meditations for building the life energy of *ki* (chi) throughout the body's meridians, becoming more emotionally balanced, focusing healing through the hands to specific areas of the body, and opening a conduit to this divine source of energy, Reiki.

Reiki Relaxation: Guided Healing Meditations. Bronwen Stiene, 2012.

This double CD offers six soothing and powerful meditations for releasing stress, clearing stuck energy, and reclaiming your ability to deeply and completely relax.

Other Animal Books

Blessing the Bridge: What Animals Teach Us About Death, Dying, and Beyond. Rita M. Reynolds. Troutdale, OR: NewSage Press, 2000.

Defending the Defenseless: A Guide to Protecting and Advocating for Pets. Allie Phillips. Lanham, MD: Rowman & Littlefield Publishers, 2011.

The Nature of Animal Healing: The Definitive Holistic Medicine Guide to Caring for Your Dog and Cat. Martin Goldstein, D.V.M. New York, NY: Ballantine Books, 2000.

Peace, Hope and Hospice: Caring for Animal Companions in Their Senior Years and Through the End of Life. Gail Pope and Lauren Urbais. BrightHaven. lulu.com. Available through lulu.com or amazon.com.

Unexpected Miracles: Hope and Holistic Healing for Pets. Shawn Messonnier, D.V.M. New York, NY: Forge Books/ Macmillan, 2009.

Spirituality

Being Peace. Thich Nhat Hanh. Berkeley, CA: Parallax Press, 2005.

Inspiration: Your Ultimate Calling. Dr. Wayne W. Dyer. Carlsbad, CA: Hay House, 2007.

A New Earth: Awakening to Your Life's Purpose by Eckhart Tolle. New York, NY: Walker and Co., 2008.

Not Always So: Practicing the True Spirit of Zen. Shunryu Suzuki. San Francisco, CA: HarperOne, 2003.

Outrageous Openness: Letting the Divine Take the Lead. Tosha Silver. Urban Kali Publishing, 2011. Available from www.toshasilver.com.

Quantum Healing: Exploring the Frontiers of Mind/Body Medicine. Deepak Choprah, M.D. New York, NY: Bantam, 1990.

The Art of Peace: Teachings of the Founder of Aikido. Morihei Ueshiba, John Stevens (Translator). Boston, MA: Shambhala, 2007.

Index

Acknowledgments

Heartfelt gratitude and thanks to:

- all the Reiki dogs of my life. You taught me how to listen.
- my human family, Che, Indigo, Maureen, John, Gini, Judy, and Kedar, and my animal family, Mystic, Shawnee, and Kodiak. You are my foundation.
- Frans Stiene, my most esteemed teacher. You inspire me.
- Leah D'Ambrosio, my dearest friend and business partner. Your love and support mean everything.
- Charlotte Jensen, my sister and editor. Your generosity and talent helped make this book a reality.
- Lexie Cataldo, photographer for this book. Thank you for sharing your special gifts.
- Kendra Luck, photographer of the cover photo. Your photo of me with Dakota will be forever precious to me.
- Gail and Richard Pope, and the animal and human family at BrightHaven. Your example is a bright light to the world.
- SARA members and my Reiki students. You are my cherished community; we are spread out so far across the world, but our hearts are one for the animals.

Acknowledgments

- Keith Reigert, Nicky Leach, and the production team at Ulysses Press. Working on this book provided so much positivity and healing for me at a very challenging time in my life health-wise. I am so grateful to be alive and be able to speak my truth. Thank you for helping me reach out to the world.

About the Author

KATHLEEN PRASAD is founder of Animal Reiki Source, offering animal Reiki treatments and instruction to animal lovers, veterinarians, vet techs, shelter and sanctuary staff, and volunteers around the world. She is also cofounder and president of the Shelter Animal Reiki Association (SARA), the first nonprofit of its kind, promoting the use of Reiki in animal shelters, sanctuaries, and rescues worldwide through treatments, education, and training programs. SARA spans the globe, with members across the U.S., Canada, England, and Australia. Kathleen has taught Reiki to the staff and volunteers of many animal organizations, including Best Friends Animal Society, the San Francisco SPCA, and Guide Dogs for the Blind.

A global leader in the profession, Kathleen has authored the profession's first animal Reiki code of ethics as well as co-authored the books *The Animal Reiki Handbook* and *Animal Reiki: Using Energy to Heal the Animals in Your Life*. She's been published in magazines such as *The Journal of the American Holistic Veterinary Medical Association*, *Dog Fancy*, and *Dogs Naturally* magazine, and has been featured in several radio and TV programs. Visit Kathleen online at www.animal reikisource.com.